Fasting Mastery:

The Ultimate Practical Guide to using Intermittent Fasting, Extended Fasting, Alternate Day, Autophagy and OMAD for Weight Loss and Optimum Health for Both Men and Women

Contents

Chapter 1: Introduction

Hello and thank you for purchasing this book. Here, we will go together into a world of nutrition and health. Of course, these two words are used so often that they become buzzwords, but this book will not be a disappointment as you shall soon see.

You may think, "Huh, another health and nutrition book that promises godlike abilities in 3 days," But the fact that you are reading this right now means that you saw the potential in this book. You might think that this one is different from the others, and you are correct. The information in this book is catered to busy people who hardly have any time to take on any new dieting tasks or cook new recipes or giving you more responsibilities. Our concern with this book is to deliver to you all the freedom, leisure, money, and most importantly, that beach body without compromising your time, health, or beauty. Yes, you heard us right. We understand that you want to lose weight and become healthier in the process. If that is what you seek, then you shall find it in this book.

You will get freedom, instead of frantically maintaining a diet and forgoing all the fun that is still left in your daily lives. You can still eat your favorite food. Of course, we will give you some suggestions on what to eat to maximize the effect of intermittent fasting, but the idea behind it is that you can go ahead with your current diet. You heard us right. You can continue to eat what you want. There is no need to cook up exotic dishes. While low-carb restriction and calorie counting can be useful but they can be quite tedious, given how busy we already are. As such, we will also cover practical tips you can follow to manage your diet without caring too much about the meticulous details.

You have many choices and can (and definitely should) enjoy your meal as usual. When you start doing intermittent fasting, you will feel healthier, less stressed, and the food that you eat will be more enjoyable.

You will have your free time, even when you are fasting. It is true that maintaining a diet cost time and transitioning to a new one costs even more. That is not the case with fasting. You do not need to spend any more time with it than you already are with your daily tasks. In fact, you will have more free time. Intermittent fasting combines normal eating with fasting, which means not eating. The time you spend not eating can be used elsewhere. You will spend less time cooking and eating, which translates to more time you could use to relax. It's just not worth cooking unhealthy food that we crave, only to regret it the day after. Moreover, you will save some money that you would on purchasing food and ingredients. You will eat less and spend less.

This book shall serve as a guide to help you get into fasting, stick to it in the most comfortable way without compromising its effectiveness. It is not a quick-fix so you will need to stick to fasting for quite some time. But hey, it doesn't consume any of your time (in fact, you will get more time from this) and the entire process is a slow, steady course to weight loss that is not only healthy but also sustainable. You will notice that you will lose a few kilos every month, and losing weight is what we ladies really care about. However, intermittent fasting is so much more than losing weight.

In this book, we will also take a look at how fasting can be beneficial for your health. You will experience two main benefits from this. First, you will be healthier because you become slimmer. You will feel better, energized, and motivated. Also, you will trigger the self-healing process in your body. That means, all the aches and pains in your body (that you slowly accept as a part of life) eventually subside without a trace.

Meanwhile, you will become even more beautiful, not in the sense of losing weight. We are talking about our skin, nails, and hair which are some of the most important things both men and women care about. They will all look better when you do intermittent fasting. Your nails will be firm, your skin will gain its elasticity, and your hair will be lush. Basically, they will have that youthful appeal once again thanks to the healing process in the body.

If you want to know more, we have included strings of numbers in our book in addition to citations from any other verified sources. The reason why we used them is the fact that it can get tedious very quickly. Many of our citations are from the National Center for Biotechnology Information, which is part of the United States National Library of Medicine where many medical journals and documents are located. You can find the documentation we cite by typing in the number such as "20339363" and then put "NCBI" on it. The first result is the document we have cited.

Do you want to find out more about how to do this intermittent fasting? Then why wait? Jump right in and let us delve deeper into this topic to a new health and nutrition trend that delivers freedom, pleasure, money, slimming, health, and beauty!

Chapter 2: Busting the Myths

Intermittent fasting and many other fasting techniques are often debated whether they are actually healthy in the long run, or if they are even effective in the first place. Moreover, myths plague the health and nutrition community, making it harder for beginners to get into the regime and get the fit body they have always wanted. Here, we will go about busting all the myths associated with fasting as a whole.

Skipping Breakfast Will Make You Fat

There is an ongoing myth saying about the importance of breakfast. You might have heard that breakfast is the most important meal of the day. People believe that they will gain weight or have cravings, or feel starving if they skip breakfast. While many studies have found that breakfast skipping and overweight or obesity are linked, it is important to note that correlation is not causation. Actually, this correlation may be explained by the fact that those who skip breakfast tend to make poor health choices as a whole. They are less health-conscious. This myth was busted recently in a randomized controlled trial, which is a sure-fire way to end all scientific disputes.

A study published in 2014 titled "The effectiveness of breakfast recommendations on weight loss: a randomized controlled trial" on NCBI compared eating breakfast versus skipping breakfast in 289 overweight and obese adults. After 16 weeks of careful observation, it was found that there was no difference in weight between groups.

So, it does not matter if you eat or do not eat breakfast in terms of weight gain, although your mileage may vary. On the other hand, some studies published on Journal of the American Dietetic Association, Volume 105, Issue 5, have shown increased performance in children and teenagers who eat breakfast, and some other studies published on the NCBI showing that those who have lost weight in the long term actually eat breakfast.

So, eating breakfast may yield benefits for many people, but it definitely is not essential. Controlled trials do not show any difference for the purpose of weight loss.

Frequent Eating Boosts Metabolism

Higher metabolism rate burns more calories, so you may think that eating many small meals would keep the flame of metabolism up. It is technically true, considering that the body also uses up the energy to consume and absorb nutrients in a meal. This is termed the thermic effect of food (TEF), and it amounts up to 20-30% of calories for protein, 5-10% for carbs, and 0-3% for fat calories. So, on average, our body uses up roughly 10% of the total calorie intake to digest food.

However, that does not mean that by eating more frequently, you can bump up your metabolism. What matters here is the total amount of calories consumed, not how frequently you eat. Let's do the math, shall we?

So, suppose that you eat six 500-calorie meals. The TEF kicks in, averaging at 10%, and you would burn 50 calories over six meals, so it would be 300 calories for those six meals. If you eat three 1000-calorie meals, then you'd get 100 calories per meal, over three meals, so you'd also burn 300 calories.

This is supported by numerous studies in human published on NCBI titled "Meal frequency and energy balance" in 1997 proving that increasing or decreasing meal frequency has no effect on total calories burned.

Frequent Meals Reduce Hunger

Some people think that snacking helps prevent cravings and excessive hunger. However, through several studies, the evidence is still mixed. While some studies have suggested that more frequent meals lead to reduced hunger, others find no effect, while others have shown to actually increased hunger levels.

Again, this is most likely the thing that varies between individuals. If snacking helps you prevent cravings and stop you from binging, then,by all means, have some snacks now and then.

Many Smaller Meals Leads to Weight Loss

We already covered the fact that frequent meal does not boost metabolism. What we have not mentioned is that they also do not seem to reduce hunger. If eating more frequently has no effect on energy consumption, then it should not have any effect on weight loss. In fact, this is supported by science. Many studies on this show that meal frequency does not affect weight loss.

Again, if you find that eating frequently helps you lower your calories intake and cut down on junk food cravings, perhaps this is effective for you. It can be very inconvenient to eat so often, but it may work for some people.

The Brain Needs a Steady Flow of Glucose

Some people believe that if they do not feed themselves with carbs every few hours, their brain will perform worse. This myth comes from the belief that the brain only uses glucose for fuel. However, what is often overlooked is the fact that the body can easily produce the glucose it needs through gluconeo genesis. In most cases, your body does not even need to do that because your body has glycogen (glucose) stored in the liver, which would be used to fuel the brain for several hours.

Even when you fast for an extended period of time, or on a very low-carb diet, the body can still produce ketone bodies from dietary fats. Ketone bodies provide energy for part of the brain, reducing its glucose needs significantly.

So, when you are on a long fast, your brain can still sustain itself using ketone bodies and glucose from proteins and fats. From an evolutionary perspective, it also makes no sense that we cannot survive without a constant source of carbohydrate. If that is true, then we would be extinct a long time ago.

However, some people feel that they are hypoglycemic when they do not eat for a while. If this is you, then maybe you should eat more frequently, but always consult your doctor before you start doing anything.

Eating and Snacking Frequently is Good for Health

Our ancestors are actually used to fast for a long time because, back then, they were hunters and gatherers. So, food does not come by as easily, and they do not last as long because they did not know how to preserve food. Since then, our body has developed to withstand starvation for a long time. It is actually not natural for us to be in a constantly fed state.

There is evidence suggesting that short-term fasting triggers a repair process in our body known as autophagy, which we will discuss in a later chapter. But basically, it is our body's way of recycling old cells and replace them with healthier ones.

The truth is, fasting now and again improves our metabolic health. Other studies have suggested that snacking, and eating often can actually damage our health and increase our risk of disease. A study found that, in addition to high-calorie intake, a diet with more frequent meals lead to a higher level of liver fat, indicating that snacking could make you more susceptible to fatty liver disease. There are also other studies showing that people who eat more frequently face a higher risk of colorectal cancer.

Fasting Puts Your Body in Starvation Mode

One thing you might have heard about fasting as a whole is that it puts your body in "starvation mode", which shuts down metabolism and stops you from burning fat. This is actually true that long-term weight loss reduces the number of calories you burn, and the actual name is adaptive thermo genesis. This can lead to up to hundreds of fewer calories burned a day.

However, this is not exclusive to fasting. Your body does this whenever you lose weight. There is no evidence suggesting that it happens more intensely with fasting than any other weight loss strategies. On the other hand, there is evidence showing that short-term fasts increase metabolic rate, caused by a drastic in blood levels of norepinephrine (noradrenaline), which signals to our fat cells to break down body fat and stimulate metabolism.

Studies have shown that fasting for up to 48 hours can boost metabolism by 3.6-10%, but if you fast any longer than that, the effect can go the opposite way and your metabolism rate goes down compared to before you start fasting. A study shows that alternative day fasting for 22 days does not decrease metabolic rate, but participants have reported that they lost about 4% of their fat mass, which is quite impressive.

The Body Can Only Burn a Certain Amount of Protein Per Meal

You may have heard from some people who said that our body can only digest 30 grams of protein each meal and that we should eat every few hours to maximize muscle gain. However, this is debunked by science yet again. Many studies which you can find on NCBI, published in 1999, 200, and 2007, have shown no difference in muscle mass if you consume protein more frequently. Just like the amount of calorie burning, what matters if the total amount, not frequency.

Intermittent Fasting Leads to Muscle Loss

Some also believe that if we fast, our bodies will start burning muscles instead of fat to fuel the body. This happens in general when you go on a diet, so this problem does not only happen when you go on intermittent fasting. In fact, some studies argued that intermittent fasting is actually better for maintaining muscle mass. In a review study on NCBI in 2011, it is found that intermittent calorie restriction yields similar weight loss result as continuous calorie restriction, but with less reduction in muscle mass.

Another study in which participants eat the same amount of calorie as they used to, except in one large dinner, shows that they lost body fat and have a slight increase (although statistically significant) in their muscle mass, along with many other beneficial effects on health markets.

In fact, intermittent fasting is very popular among bodybuilders, who view it as an effective way to maintain high amounts of muscle with a low body fat percentage.

Intermittent Fasting is Unhealthy

Some people are led to believe that fasting is harmful, but it is false. Many studies show that intermittent fasting, and intermittent calorie restriction, can lead to many health benefits. For instance, intermittent fasting has been shown to prolong lifespan in test animals because it changes the expression of genes related to longevity and disease. It is also great for metabolic health, such as greater insulin sensitivity, lowered oxidative stress and inflammation, ad lowered risk factors for heart disease.

It may also be great for brain health as fasting boosts levels of a brain hormone called brain-derived neurotrophic factor (BDNF), which can protect you from depression and other brain problems.

Intermittent Fasting Leads to Overeating

This is probably one of the things you would be told if you say that you are considering fasting for weight loss. They may say something like, "Well, if you intentionally starve yourself, wouldn't you eat more than you should after you fast?" This is one of the things you may hear, as they often claim that fasting will not lead to weight loss as it causes you to overeat during the eating period to compensate for the lack of nutrition you subjected yourself to earlier.

This is partially true because people tend to eat a little more after fasting. In other words, they try to compensate for the calories lost during the fast by eating more during the next few meals or so. However, you should know that this compensation is not complete. A study on NCBI in 2002 titled "Effect of an acute fast on energy compensation and feeding behavior in lean men and women" showed that people who fasted for 24 hours only eat 500 calories the next day. Here, the participants expended about 2,400 calories during the fast and then overate by 500 calories the next day. The total reduction in calorie intake was then 1,900 calories, which is a huge drop.

Intermittent fasting also reduces overall food intake while boosting your metabolism. It reduces insulin levels, increases norepinephrine and boosts hormones related to human growth up to five times. Because of these effects, intermittent fasting actually makes you lost fat, not gain it.

According to a 2014 review study, fasting between 3 to 24 weeks causes body weight loss of 3-8%, and 4-7% decrease in belly fat. Here, intermittent fasting led to 0.55 pounds of weight loss a week, but alternating-day fasting led to 1.65 pounds of weight loss a week.

Final Verdict

So, really, there is nothing unhealthy about fasting as a whole. If you wish to lose weight, then fasting is the way to go. The fact is, intermittent fasting is one of the best tools you can utilize to lose weight. You may think that depriving yourself of food for a while every day is unnatural. Some people share the same view, and they argue that humans survive because they eat. While that is true but you should know that there is nothing wrong or unnatural about fasting. Humans have been doing it for thousands of years, mainly out of necessity because there simply wasn't any food available. In some other cases, fasting is done for religious reasons. Islam, Christianity, and Buddhism introduce some form of fasting. Therefore, our body well adapted to fasting from time to time.

Therefore, our body is actually prepared to go on extended periods of starvation. The problem here is that we tend to feed it regularly, but it does not tell our body that we now live in abundance. Your body is always on high alert and so it tries to stock up as much as possible to prepare for the time of starvation that never comes. As such, we pack on weight. Fasting allows us to burn that energy reserve and maintain our health.

Chapter 3: Which Fasting Is For You?

In this chapter, we will look at all kinds of fasting and discuss them in details so you know which one works for you. There are many kinds of fasting out there, some of which are safe whereas others are not. We will focus on common methods and how to do them.

16/8

16/8 intermittent fasting is the most basic and practiced form of IF. Here, you need to fast for 16 hours and use the remaining 8 hours to eat, hence the name.

You should adhere to the 16/8 method and its hours, but you do not need to count the seconds. This method is best for beginners as it is very easy to do. However, you may have difficulties with this method at first, especially during that time of the month, and my lady coworkers also said that they had trouble as well. If you have trouble adapting to the 16/8 method, you can alter it a bit. We sometimes fast for only 14 hours and eat within the 10-hour window. 16/10 is not as effective, but it is good enough during the hard times. Plus, the body still has enough time to clean itself.

The main reason why this method is preferred, even among IF veterans, is the fact that you will still receive enough food every day. It is not that you will starve for a long time. You will spend about half of the fasting period sleeping if you sleep for 8 hours a day (and you should). Everyone could do with one less meal for a day.

I have a good tip for you. Eating the right food helps. You should eat high-fat food or eggs as the last meal before fasting. If you eat something sweet, then the food is quickly turned into glucose. In your body, this means that the blood sugar level rises rapidly. As a result, your body releases insulin and the blood sugar level drops again, but it will also drop below its normal value, and then you quickly have another craving for sweets.

In the end, if you eat some greasy or eggs, then your stomach and your intestines will take longer to digest. This gives you a long feeling of being full. Then you are hungry and can easily survive fasting.

How you arrange the hours of fasting is entirely up to you, only 16 (or 14) hours must be in one piece. There are several possible combinations. Let's say you drop the breakfast. Then your first meal of the day is your lunch, and you have it at 12. Then you eat something smaller like coffee, then you have dinner at 8. Then, eat eggs or something fried, and you go to bed a few hours later. In the morning, you get up, skip breakfast, drink some coffee, water or tea, and then go to work. But we advise against drinking coffee because if you drink too much, your body will become overstimulated and you will feel hungry.

If you stick to this routine, you will find that you have a lot of energy in the morning and do not really feel any craving for food. Then, before you know it, it's already noon, and you can enjoy your lunch. Then congratulations, because you have just survived 16 hours of fasting.

If you prefer to eat in the morning, you can still be flexible with your time. So you can start fasting at 3 in the afternoon and then stop at 7 o'clock in the morning the next day, and start the day with breakfast. After breakfast, you have lunch at 12 o'clock.

As we said, the time of fasting and eating are not set in stone, and you are free to make your own rules completely. So you can also start fasting at 4pm or 10pm and then stop later. The important thing is that you fast at least 14 hours, better still 16, and once you've found your favorite time, you should stick to it. By maintaining a fixed rhythm, you allow your body to get used to it, so you will soon no longer be hungry by itself.

During fasting, however, you must always make sure to drink enough for fast to succeed. You should definitely avoid alcohol, sweet drinks and the like. Have unsweetened tea and water and a cup of coffee. Then you will soon realize how much better you are.

Now it can happen that one or the other is a little bit hard to get into this method of fasting immediately. Here it is possible to slowly get used to the fasting. In such a case, you should first decide what times you want to choose for fasting and which times you want to eat. Let's say you want to fast from 8pm to 12pm. In this case, you start having breakfast always a little later. You usually eat at 7 o'clock, then you move it to 7:30 o'clock. At the same time, you are putting lunch a little bit ahead. So you bring the two meals closer together until they overlap. Then move that eating time slowly to lunch time and voila, you are now in your 16 to 8 rhythm.

Crescendo Method

If you do a quick Google search of intermittent fasting for women, you will find that the crescendo method is the best for them. It works in unison with their lady hormones. This method is a gentle way to get women into intermittent fasting, which is perfect for ladies. It doesn't rub their hormones in the wrong way.

The main reason why it is great for ladies and beginners alike is the fact that it is realistic. You do not need to fast for 16 hours a day. 12 hours is good enough. You can have dinner at 8 PM and breakfast at 8 AM, it's like a normal day. You fast for 12 hours. It is easy to get into this routine.

But do you know what else we like about this method?

You do not have to fast on a daily basis. You can be flexible with the days you want to spend fasting. You just need to spend a few non-consecutive days of fasting every week, and you are good to go! So, you can eat normally on a Monday because Monday is horrible and you want to make it as least horrible as possible. Then, you do that again on Wednesday. Then, you eat normally on a Friday because you might want to enjoy your Friday night and the weekend. You fast for 12 hours on Tuesday, Thursday, Saturday, and Sunday. Voila! You have a perfect week.

Even though this method of fasting is gentle, it is still shown that it can reduce body fat, lessen inflammation, and improve your energy.

There are some tips we would like to give you to help you get into the routine. First, you should alternate the days you fast. Try not to have consecutive eating days like Monday to Wednesday and then fast for the rest of the week. You might feel horrible at the end of the week. Some people fast on Tuesday, Thursday, and Saturday, but we found that fasting on Monday, Wednesday, and Friday works the best for me. Still, it's worth experimenting and sticks to what works best for you. Again, try not to have consecutive fasting days.

On those fasting days, try to squeeze in some lower intensity workout, if you do exercise (and you probably should). We will discuss how exercise can be useful for intermittent fasting in a later chapter. It is also worth mentioning that you should eat healthy food every day, get in enough water, about 64 ounces, every day.

Now, if you are starting out and are unsure about this whole fasting method, you can start small. Start with 1 day of fasting a week, then bump it up to 2 and then 3 when you are ready.

Eat, Stop, Eat or OMAD

Eat, stop, eat (ESE) aka OMAD (one meal a day) method is also a commonly used method. This method was founded by Brad Pilon who thought of the plan when he was doing his graduate research on short-term fasting at the University of Guelph. Basically, you fast once a twice a week, but you need to fast for 24 hours at a time. Then, on the other days, you can eat as much as you want, as long as you eat responsibly, that is. Brad wrote that he is okay with whatever eating pattern you adopt, so long as you eat responsibly and it works for you.

Still, he advises against not eating for the entire day. You should schedule your time in a way that you can have a meal every day, and still fast in-between. That means you should not fast from midnight on Monday to midnight on Tuesday. Instead, have dinner at 8 on a Monday and fast until dinnertime at 8 on a Tuesday. That way, you still eat something every day and fast at the same time. You need that energy to get through the day, after all.

Because ESE method is different from the previous two methods since you need to not eat for 24 hours, it is worth looking into how it works. According to Eliza Whetzel-Savage, R.D., a registered dietitian with Middleburg Nutrition in NYC, when you reduce the eating window, you create a larger fasting period during which the body will use the stored glycogen from carbohydrates as well as fat to fuel the body. When glycogen and glucose are burnt up, your body goes into a ketogenic state and then burn fat for fuel. This basically translates to you losing weight. The ESE method is simply a twist to the existing IF methods by extending the periods of fasting and eating, and it works just as well as the other method.

Because ESE method requires you to go on a long stretch of fasting, you should expect it to have its own upside and downside, so you decide if you want to try it.

The upside is the fact that you only restrict your calorie intake once or twice a week or every other day. For the rest of the week, you can eat however you want, within reasons of course. You should still eat nutritious foods when you break your fast. You can be flexible with your time frame, meaning that you can start fasting at 6 in the morning or 10 in the evening – whatever works best for you. Then, you start eating 24 hours later. Of course, you should time it so that you at least have a meal every day.

Because you need to fast only once or twice a week, you can fit it into your life very easily along with other routines like a workout, parties, work, family, etc. Moreover, you do not necessarily have to starve yourself for 24 hours. You can help yourself with some green tea (0 cals) or black coffee (3 cals), and have some solid food such as an egg or an apple during the day. This is done so that you would not black out from the absolute lack of food. Let's face it. Our bodies are different anyway, so it's worth ensuring your safety when you go on this diet regime if your mileage varies. The ESE method is probably for you if you want to try something different. It is easy for beginners as well because they just need to focus on fasting once or twice a week. If you fast during the days that you are very busy, then you might focus less on your own hunger. Otherwise, you can fast on a weekend day because you do not need as much energy if you stay in. You can rest to compensate for the lack of food, and you can distract yourself from the hunger with things you like to do.

At the same time, however, you should be aware of some downsides. Of course, not eating 24 hours at a time can be tough for some people and it can actually increase the likelihood of bingeing when the fasting is over, which defeats the purpose of fasting. There is no point in restricting your calorie intake once or twice a week if you are just going to compensate for the loss of calorie by overeating for the rest of the week.

The ESE method works only if you are willing to go the long stretch of fasting at a time, and can control yourself from not overeating for the rest of the week. It might not be for you if you often need to go out with your friends and family very often. Another thing that we should point out is that, if you have any medical complications with fasting, we advise you to talk to your doctor before you start any new eating plan, including intermittent fasting.

While OMAD requires you to restrict your calorie intake for almost 24 hours at a time, it is worth pointing out that it will not work if you do not control what you eat. You may be surprised to know that all that 23 hours of progress will be for naught if you eat uncontrollably for that one-hour window. So, what do you need when you are on the ESE diet?

Food to Eat

For veggies, you should eat kale, spinach, white potato with peek, sweet potato, bell peppers, lettuce, Chinese cabbage, purple cabbage, scallions, turnip, beetroot, cauliflower, cabbage, broccoli, and carrot.

For fruits, you should eat acai berries, gooseberries, blueberries, strawberries, pineapple, tangerine, lime, lemon, plum, peach, tomato, cucumber, grapes, grapefruit, orange, banana, apple, and a limited number of mangoes.

For your protein fix, your options include eggs, tofu, beans and legumes, mushroom, fish, lean cuts of pork and beef, and chicken breast.

As for your diary, you can choose from cottage cheese, homemade ricotta cheese, buttermilk, feta cheese, cheddar cheese, full-fat yogurt, and full-fat milk.

As for fats and oils, you have almond butter, peanut butter, sunflower butter, olive oil, rice bran oil, and edible grade coconut oil.

If you love eating nuts and seeds, you can eat melon seeds, pumpkin seeds, sunflower seeds, macadamia, pistachios, pine nuts, pecan, almond, and walnut.

As for herbs and spices, you have clove, garlic powder, cardamom, star anise, allspice, chili flakes, white pepper, black pepper, cayenne pepper, turmeric, cumin, coriander, onion, ginger, garlic, oregano, thyme, rosemary, fennel, dill, mint, and cilantro.

Finally, for something to wet your mouth, you can go for water, homemade lemonade or electrolyte, coconut water, cold-pressedjuices,and freshly pressed fruit juice.

As you can probably tell, you are already spoiled for choices here even when you undertake this ESE fasting method. In fact, you can even implement these into your other fasting regime because the selection above is all very healthy for you. With these, you can cook up some delectable dishes for yourself as a reward for your hard work. Of course, these are generally what you should eat. We also want to point out some of the things you need to avoid to maintain your health.

What Not to Eat

When it comes to fruit, you need to avoid fruits rich in GI such as grapes, jackfruit, pineapples, and mangoes. You can eat them but limit your intake.

As for protein, avoid fatty cuts of beef and pork, and bacon (especially bacon).

For dairy products, avoid low-fat milk, low-fat yogurt, cream cheese, and flavored yogurt.

You should also avoid whole grains such as white rice. Consume it in limited quantity and always eat it with at least five other veggies in the previous list to balance it out with the GI.

For fat and oils, avoid mayonnaise, margarine, butter, vegetable oil, lard, dalda, and hemp seed oil.

For nuts and seeds, avoid cashew nuts like the plague.

Also, avoid processed foods such as salami, ranch dip, sausages, fries, jellies, and bottled jams.

As for beverages, avoid packaged fruit and vegetable juices, soda, diet soda (it doesn't help), and energy drinks.

Now that you know what to avoid, let us discuss how you could design your meal so that you do not lose your head while on the ESE diet.

What to Include in Your Meal

- Five types of veggies
- Three types of fruits
- Lean protein, but you can eat some red meat once in a while

- Lots of plant protein like kidney beans, seeds, nuts, garbanzo beans, and whole pulses (if you are a vegetarian)
- A cup of buttermilk or half a bowl of curd to help digest food
- A few unsalted nuts, only a few
- A piece of 80% dark chocolate, if you need to
- Fruits, sour cream, or yogurt if you want some more sweet treats
- Alternatively, you can bake and store brownies that have healthy ingredients and less sugar
- Keep yourself hydrated – you limit your calorie intake, not your fluid intake; stay well hydrated as this is one of the only things that keep you going
- Alternatively, you can drink three or four cups of green tea during your fasting period
- If you exercise, make sure you have an egg before you start and replenish your electrolyte reserve by drinking coconut water after you are done

We will talk more about exercise in a later chapter, but you may already be wondering if you should consider working out when you are on this strict dieting regime. After all, you do not eat for almost 24 hours, so surely you would feel tired at the end of the day – both mentally and physically. Exercising would only push yourself further, you may argue. Well, let's talk about this.

ESE and Exercise

At first, when you fast for an extended period of time, your body will need to adjust and so you may feel exhausted, unable to exercise. This is normal. Even if you attempt to exercise, the fatigue may weaken you so much that you cannot put enough effort into doing it properly, which could result in serious injuries in some cases. Your body has not been fed for a long time, and so your muscles are also weakened. To keep your muscles active, start light by doing stretching exercises or yoga first.

From there, as your body starts to adjust to the new eating routine, you can slowly introduce muscle toning workouts to prevent the sagging of your skin. Of course, you should always consult a qualified and competent trainer to design a workout that suits you, while accounting for your medical condition and body type. Whether you go on the ESE diet or not, you should always practice meditation everyday through the traditional method, or when you are out walking or running.

Risks and Cautions

There are a few things you need to know if you are just starting out. Even when you are used to the 16/8 method, extending your fasting period to almost 24 hours and leaving yourself with a little room to eat can be tricky still.

When you first start this diet plan, you will feel hungry and restless. Do not panic. This is natural. You may feel dizzy and experience brain fog along the way too, especially toward the end of your fasting phase. You might not be able to concentrate properly and metabolism in menopausal women may slow down.

Because our bodies respond differently to the same diets, it is absolutely necessary that you consult your doctor or a registered dietitian before you start following this diet. Moreover, pregnant or lactating women should not try this diet.

Alternate-Day Fasting

Alternate-day fasting is yet another fasting approach and an alteration to the OMAD/ESE method. Here, the idea is that you fast for one day, eat normally the next, and fast again the next day. On fasting days, you can drink as many calorie-free beverages as you want, such as water, unsweetened coffee, and tea.

If this is too hard for you, you can use a modified ADF approach by eating only 500 calories on fasting days, or only 20-25% of your energy requirements. It seems that the weight loss benefits are the same regardless of whether you consume calories at lunch, dinner, or as small meals throughout the day. As always, your mileage may vary so you may find that one of the previous methods work better for you than ADF. Because you get to consume something during the fasting day to keep your body going, the modified version of ADF is a lot more sustainable than doing full fasts on fasting days and it is just as effective anyway.

Health Benefits

Other than weight loss, ADF has many health benefits such as:

Type 2 Diabetes

Type 2 diabetes accounts for 95% of diabetes cases in the United States. To make matter worse, more than a third of Americans are obese and have pre-diabetes, a condition in which their blood sugar levels are higher than normal but not high enough to be considered diabetes. A great way to improve your health and reverse many debilitating symptoms of type 2 diabetes is by losing weight and restricting calories.

Just like continuous calorie restriction, ADF causes a mild reduction in risk factors associated with type 2 diabetes among overweight and obese individuals. However, this fasting method is the most effective in lowering insulin levels and reducing insulin resistance with only a small effect on blood sugar control, which is amazing considering that having high insulin levels have been linked to obesity and other chronic diseases such as cancer and heart disease. Only 8 to 12 weeks have been shown to decrease fasting insulin by about 30% among pre-diabetic individuals.

Overall, the reduction in insulin levels and insulin resistance lead to reduced risk of type 2 diabetes, especially when you lose weight in the process.

Heart Health

Heart disease is one of the leading cause of death in the world, responsible for about 1 in 4 deaths. This is one of the worst ways to go too, considering that it could strike at any time, and there are little you can do to prepare yourself for it. Many studies have shown that ADF is a good option for obese and overweight individuals to lose weight so they can reduce heart disease risk factors. Many studies on the subject range from 8 to 12 weeks of ADF and their subjects are overweight and obese individuals. The most common health benefits you can get from ADF include:

- Decreased blood pressure
- Lower LDL cholesterol concentration (20-25%)
- Decreased blood triglycerides (Up to 30%)
- Decreased blood pressure
- Increase number of large LDL-particles and reduction in dangerous small, dense LDL particles
- Reduced waist circumference (5-7cm or 2-2.9in)

Alternate-Day Fasting and Autophagy

ADF also has a special interaction with autophagy, which we will get to in a later chapter. ADF stimulates autophagy, which is a process in which old parts of your cells are recycled and replaced with better ones. So, your body can prevent diseases such as cancer, neuro degeneration, heart disease, and other infections. Studies on animals have shown that both long-term and short-term fasting increase autophagy. Plus, they linked to a delay in aging and reduced risk of tumors.

Moreover, fasting has also been shown to increase lifespan in rodents, flies, yeasts, and worms. As far as we know, human studies have shown that ADF does reduce oxidative damage and promote changes that may be linked to longevity. Of course, you should not expect that you will live longer by a significant margin, but you can take comfort in knowing that at least you will live healthier with ADF.

ADF and Starvation Mode

Most weight loss methods cause a slight drop in resting metabolic rate, and high metabolic rate is what we want to maintain here. This drop is known as the starvation mode, but the technical term is adaptive thermogenesis.

When you restrict your calories, your body will attempt to conserve energy by reducing the number of calories it burns. Your body does not necessarily need to burn the same amount of calories every day in order to function. Think of it as the battery saving mode. You may feel a bit sluggish, but you do not tire as quickly. However, that is the problem. When your body does not burn as many calories, you stop losing weight while also making you feel miserable. Here, ADF does not seem to cause a drop in metabolic rate.

There was a study that compared ADF to standard calorie restriction over eight weeks, and the results showed that continuous calorie restriction causes a significant drop in resting metabolic rate by 6%, whereas ADF only causes a small dip of 1%. Moreover, after 24 unsupervised weeks, the subjects that underwent standard calorie restriction still had a 4.5% lower resting metabolic rate compared to before the study, whereas the ADF subjects maintained their original metabolic rate. Many effects associated with ADF may be responsible for maintaining a relatively high metabolic rate, including the preservation of muscle mass.

Is It Good for Normal-Weight People?

ADF has its uses outside weight-loss. It also has many health benefits even for normal-weight people. A 3-week study conducted on individuals with normal-weight who follow a strict ADF diet, with zero calories on fasting days, showed increased fat burning rate, decreased fasting insulin rate, and a 4% decrease in fat mass. However, subjects reported that they felt hungry throughout the study. That is why you should consider following the ADF diet with one small meal on fasting days, as it is more tolerable for normal-weight people.

Another controlled study on both normal-weight and overweight individuals showed that, after following ADF diet for 12 weeks, resulted in reduced fat mass and favorable changes in risk factors associated with heart disease. Here, it is worth pointing out that the reason why you lose weight is the fact that ADF normally gives you much fewer calories than you need to maintain weight. If you do not want to lose weight or fat mass in the first place, then ADF may not be for you, and other dietary methods will most likely suit you better.

Drinks

There is no general rule when it comes to what you should eat or drink on fasting days, except that it should not exceed 500 calories in total. So, it is best to drink low or calorie-free drinks on fasting days, such as water, coffee, and tea. Many people find it best to eat a large meal late in the day, while others prefer eating early or split the meal between 2 to 3 meals, all within 500 calories.

Because your calorie intake will be limited, you should make sure you get the 500 calories from nutritious, high-protein foods, as well as low-calorie vegetables. That way, you will feel full without consuming too many calories. You should also consider trying out soups because they tend to make you feel fuller than if you eat the ingredients separately.

Here are a few ideas of what you should eat during fasting days:

- Lots of salad with lean meat
- Soup and piece of fruit
- Grilled fish or lean meat with vegetables
- Yogurt with berries
- Eggs and vegetables

There are also plenty of quick 500-calorie meals and healthy low-calorie snacks out there. All you need is a quick Google search. As always, make sure to check if you have any allergies to any of the ingredients. You do not want to have a nasty surprise while you are fasting.

Is it Safe?

The final verdict. According to numerous studies, ADF is shown to be safe for most people. Quite contrary to belief, ADF does not result in a greater risk of weight regain compared to traditional, calorie-restricted diets. On the other hand, ADF may be better for long-term weight loss compared to continuous calorie restriction.

Some believe that ADF heightens risks of overeating or binge eating, but studies have shown that it actually decreased depression and binge eating. It also improved restrictive eating and body image perception among obese individuals.

Of course, we said that ADF is shown to be safe with most people is because there are always groups of people who should not adhere to any weight loss diet. So, consult your doctor before you start changing up your diet plans, especially if you have a medical condition or are currently taking any medications. These groups include people with eating disorders, pregnant and lactating mothers, children and underweight individuals or those who have certain medical conditions.

The 5:2 Diet aka "Fast Diet"

The 5:2 diet, which is also known as the Fast Diet, is one of the easiest fasting diets. Popularized by British Journalist Michael Mosely, this diet got its name because you will get five days a week eating normally and the other two are restricted to 500-600 calories a day. Similar to a few other intermittent fasting methods, what matters here is when you eat your meals, not what you eat. So, this is more of a lifestyle than a diet regimen. A lot of people find that this is easier than a traditional calorie-restricted diet.

It is very simple to follow. You fast for 2 nonconsecutive days and consume 500 calories if you are a woman, and 600 calories if you are a man. What days you fast do not matter, just make sure that there is at least one non-fasting day in between them.

If losing weight is your priority, then the 5:2 diet can prove to be very effective if done properly. This is because the 5:2 method helps you consume fewer calories without putting too much stress on your body. The weight loss comes when you fast for those two days, and the lack of calorie will force your body to consume the fat in your body while still providing enough so that your body does not eat up your muscles or slowing down metabolism to preserve energy. Because you will only lose weight during the two fasting days, it is critical that you do not compensate for the calories you missed during the fasting day by eating more on non-fasting days.

This method will not work if you compensate for the calories you missed. That said, fasting methods similar to the 5:2 diet have shown a lot of promise in weight loss studies:

- A recent review discovered that modified alternate-day fasting led to weight loss of 3 to 8% over 3 to 24 weeks.
- In the same study, participants have reported that their waist circumference has shrunk by 4 to 7%, meaning that they have lost a lot of harmful belly fat.
- Intermittent fasting causes a significant reduction in muscle mass compared to other weight loss with conventional calorie restriction.
- Combined with exercises, intermittent fasting is even more effective, such as endurance or strength training. We will discuss this in more details later.

How to Eat on Fasting Days

There is no role for what or when you should eat on fasting days here, unlike the 16:8 method. Some people find it more convenient when they start their day with a small breakfast.

Others find that eating as late as possible is better. Normally though, there are two meals pattern that people follow.

You can have three meals a day as usual, but the amount of calorie is divided between those three meals. So, if you are a man, you can divide your 600 calories over three meals. You'd have 200 calories for breakfast, lunch, and dinner equally. That, or you could have a 300-calorie breakfast, 200-calorie lunch, and 100-calorie dinner. Again, it is up to you to decide how you want to portion your limited number of calories throughout the day, although it may be a good idea to start off strong with a relatively large breakfast, smaller lunch, and smallest dinner as you may not need to spend as much energy at the end of the day. The same applies if you are a woman, although you will only have 500 calories to work it so divide them wisely. You can have somewhat balanced meals of 250-calorie breakfast, 150-calorie lunch, and 150-calorie dinner. That or prioritize getting most out of your breakfast with 300-calorie breakfast, and 100-calorie lunch and dinner. Again, experiment and find out what works best for you and stick to it.

Another approach is to have two slightly larger meals instead of three. The same principle applies, except that you can only get to eat twice. Whatever you do, remember that your calorie intake is limited – 600 for men and 500 for women. So, it is best to use your calorie budget wisely. It is best to make the most out of your calorie intake, so we suggest that you go for nutritious, high-fiber, high-protein foods that make you feel full without consuming too many calories. As mentioned previously, soups are a great option. A few examples of healthy foods include:

- Still or sparkling water
- Tea
- Black coffee
- Low-calorie cup soups
- Soups (miso, tomato, cauliflower or vegetables)
- A generous amount of vegetables
- Boiled or baked eggs
- Grilled fish or lean meat
- Natural yogurt with berries
- Cauliflower rice

Again, there are no one-size-fits-all meals here, so you need to experiment a bit to find out what works for you and stick to it.

Feeling Unwell?

If you are new to fasting and intermittent fasting, expect to experience moments of overwhelming hunger. This is normal. You may also feel weaker or slower than usual. However, hunger will eventually fade, especially if you try to distract yourself with work or other errands. Moreover, fasters reported that the fasting regimen gets easier after the first few fasts. You certainly are going to be alright.

However, there is no need to torture yourself if it gets unbearable. So, if you are not used to fasting, it may be a good idea to keep some small snack handy during your first few fasts, just in case you feel faint or ill.

However, if you continue to feel ill or faint during fast days, eat something and consult with your doctor about whether you should continue. Fasting is not for everyone, and some people cannot tolerate it. Of course, fasting is very safe or healthy, but as we have mentioned time and again, your mileage may vary. It does not suit everyone. It is more intended for healthy, well-nourished individuals. Some people should avoid fasting or any other dietary restrictions completely, including:

- Pregnant women, nursing mothers, teenagers, children and people with type 1 diabetes
- Individuals who often experience drops in sugar levels
- Individuals with a history of eating disorders
- Individuals who are malnourished, underweight, or have known nutrient deficiencies
- Women who have fertility issues or are trying to conceive

Water Fasting

Another form of fasting is known as water fasting, which restricts anything but water. It has been an effective way to lose weight as well. Some studies (19818847) have shown that water fasting could yield some health benefits. It can lower the risk of some chronic diseases and might stimulate autophagy, which is the way your body recycles. However, it is worth pointing out that there are only a few studies conducted on human, and water fasting also has many health risks, therefore making it unsuitable for some people.

Most water fasts last between 24 to 72 hours, and if you wish to carry on any longer than that, you need medical supervision. There are some reasons why people try out water fasting:

- For its health benefits
- Preparing for a medical procedure

- For detoxing
- For weight loss
- Religious or spiritual reasons

The reason why we put health benefits up there is that several studies have found many impressive health benefits associated with water fastings, such as a lower risk of cancer, diabetes, and heart disease (PMC3106288, 19818847, PMC4509734), in addition to promoting autophagy.

Dangers and Risks of Water Fasting

In reality, popular diets such as the lemon detox cleanse are modeled after water fasting because it only permits drinking a combination of lemon juice, water, maple syrup, and cayenne pepper, many times a day for a week. However, if you follow water fasting for far too long, it may be very dangerous for your body.

Wrong Weight Loss

Because water has zero calories, you will lose a lot of weight very quickly. In fact, each day of the 24- to 72-hour water fast, you may lose up to 2 pounds or almost a kilo (6758355). However, the weight you lose may come from the water in your body, carbs, or even muscle mass.

Dehydration

Okay, it sounds strange to say that water fasting leads to dehydration. The reason why it happens is thatroughly 20-30% of the water you consume come from the food you eat. If you drink the same amount of water but not eat food, you might not get enough water still. A general rule is that you should drink about 2 liters or half a gallon of water a day, but you may need to drink more water if you go on a water fast. You know that you are not getting enough water when you experience dizziness, headaches, nausea, constipation, low blood pressure, and low productivity.

Orthostatic Hypotension

People who water fast usually experience orthostatic hypotension, which is defined as a drop in blood pressure that occurs when you stand up suddenly. When that happens, you may experience dizziness, lightheadedness, and a small risk of fainting altogether. If you are suffering from orthostatic hypotension when you fast, you should avoid driving or operating heavy machinery as the symptoms may lead to an accident. Moreover, you should stop waterfasting immediately. Drop whatever you are doing, sit or lie down, grab a bite or two and rest.

Worsened Medical Conditions

While a water fast may not last as long, a few conditions may be worsened by water fasting. Therefore, you should avoid water fasting without first consulting with a doctor if you have the following medical condition:

- Heartburn: Fasting may cause heartburn, because your body may continue to make stomach acid without any food to digest
- Eating disorders: There is some evidence suggesting that fasting may encourage eating disorders especially in teenagers (PMC2850570)
- Chronic kidney disease: Water fasting might damage the kidneys in people with this disease
- Diabetes: Fasting might also increase the risk of the nasty side effects in type 1 and type 2 diabetes
- Gout: Water fasting may also increase the production of uric acid, which is a risk factor of gout attacks

Benefits of Water Fasting

On the other hand, water fasting has also been linked to many health benefits in humans and animal studies.

Autophagy

As mentioned previously, autophagy is our body's way of recycling and it can prevent diseases such as cancer, Alzheimer's disease, as well as heart disease. In the case of cancer, autophagy finds cells that are damaged and replace parts of it so the cell can function as new. The prevention of this error from accumulating can stop cancer from growing.

Research conducted on animals also consistently find that water fasting help promote autophagy and it may help extend lifespan as well (PMC2696814). That said, there are not enough studies on humans to confidently assert that water fasting, autophagy, and disease prevention.

Lower Blood Pressure

Medically supervised water fasts that last longer than 72 hours may lead to lowered blood pressure for those who have high blood pressure. In a study, 68 people who have high blood pressure followed water fasting for almost 14 days under close medical supervision. In the end, 82% of the participants had significantly reduced blood pressure to a healthy level (12470446).

In another study, 174 people with high blood pressure followed water fasting routing for an average of 10 to 11 days, and at the end of the fast, 90% of them achieved a blood pressure lower than 140/90 mmHg, which is the limit used to diagnose high blood pressure (11416824).

Better Insulin and Leptin Sensitivity

Insulin and leptin are important hormones that affect your metabolism rate. Insulin helps the body store nutrients from the bloodstream and leptin reduce your appetite by making you feel full. Research shows that water fasting has the potential to make your body more sensitive to these two hormones. Greater sensitivity means that the hormones are more effective (PMC156352, 25912765).

For instance, when your body is more sensitive to insulin, it is more efficient in reducing blood sugar. Higher sensitivity to leptin means that your body process hunger signals more efficiently, meaning that it can tell when you feel full more accurately, which can lower your risk of obesity.

Lowered Risk of Chronic Diseases

There is some evidence that water fasting might lower the risk of chronic diseases such as diabetes, cancer, and heart disease (22323820, 10524500). In a study, 30 healthy adults water fasted for 24 hours. Results showed that they had significantly lower blood levels of cholesterol and triglycerides, which are the two risk factors for heart disease (23220077).

Many experiments conducted on animals also showed that water fasting could protect the heart against damage from free radicles, which are unstable molecules that can damage parts of the cells and are known to cause many chronic diseases. Moreover, water fasting may suppress genes that help cancer cells grow, meaning that it could make chemotherapy more effective.

How to Water Fast

There is no main science-based guideline on how to start water fasting. As mentioned earlier, water fasting is not compatible with many kinds of people, and you should prepare your body a few days in advance before you attempt to water fast. You can do this by eating smaller and smaller portions of food at each meal or by fasting for several hours a day.

Water fast means that you cannot drink or eat anything other than water. As a general rule, you should drink two to three liters of water a day, and you should only fast like this for at most 72 hours. Any longer would put you at great health risk. If you want to fast any longer, seek medical supervision. You may feel weak or dizzy during a water fast and should avoid operating heavy machinery and driving to avoid causing accidents.

After the fast, your body is still too frail to handle a big meal. As tempting as it may be, refrain from eating a big meal. Eating a large meal right after a water fast may cause uncomfortable symptoms. Instead, we suggest that you break your fast with a smoothie or smaller meals. You can work your way up from there.

The post-fast phase is also important after long fasts because you are at risk of the refeeding syndrome, which is a potentially fatal condition where the body undergoes rapid changes in fluid and electrolytes. The post-fast phase usually lasts 24 hours, but if you fast for 72 hours, then you may need up to three days before you feel comfortable eating larger meals again.

Water Fasting and Fat Burning

Unfortunately, water fasting is not a good way to burn fat. It can help you lose weight rapidly, but you will most likely lose water weight, carbs, and muscle mass rather than fat. Moreover, water fasts may pose health risks that can be avoided easily. That is why we suggest that you try intermittent fasting or alternate-day fasting rather than a water fast unless water fasting works way better than the previous two methods of fasting.

Intermittent Fasting and Its Effects

Intermittent fasting is the current health and fitness trends. Many people talk about it. Many people claim that they have a lot of benefits, while some say otherwise. Perhaps you are familiar with it. Many people are using it to lose weight, improve their health, all within their own convenience. Numerous studies have shown that intermittent fasting can have powerful effects on your body and brain, not to mention that it may even improve your longevity. So, what is intermittent fasting?

Intermittent fasting, IF for short, involves alternating cycles of fasting and eating. That's it. It is more of a pattern of eating than a diet. You simply schedule your meals so that you can get the most out of them. IF does not change what you eat. It alters when you do so.

Many studies show that IF can help you lose weight, improve your metabolic health, strengthen your immune system and improve your longevity. We will look deeper into the science behind intermittent fasting and the benefits in later chapters.

Because IF is an alternating eat-fast pattern, there are many methods for IF and the most notable difference is when you should and should not eat. The best thing about IF is that it is an amazing way to get lean without going on a crazy diet you found on the internet or cutting your calorie down to almost zero, making you feel starved and tired all the time. Let's face it, ladies, we need a solution that is easy to stick to. Sure, IF will take a while before you can see the benefits, but we won't be torturing ourselves in the process.

Commonly, there are two methods of fasting, the 16/8, which means fasting for 16 hours and eat for 8 hours, and the OMAD/ESE method in which you fast for 24 hours at a time, twice a week. There are also other variations of intermittent fasting as well, and we will get to them later.

When you think about it, we are already fasting every day. We do it when we sleep. When you look at it that way, intermittent fasting is as simple as skipping breakfast. If you do that, then you are already practicing the 16/8 method of IF (methods to be discussed in a later chapter). Allow me to explain. Suppose that you eat lunch at 12 and dinner at 8, then when you skip breakfast, you are already limiting your eating window into the 8-hour period between lunch and dinner. If you do not eat anything else outside that period, then you would be fasting for 16 hours. It can just be that simple!

Now, if you are unfamiliar with IF, you may think that it is difficult and unhealthy. It is true that skipping a meal may seem counterintuitive, but it is actually very easy to do, and many people are already reporting that they feel better and have more energy when they fast. Skipping a meal, resulting in hunger, is not that big of a deal either. It can be a problem in the beginning because your body is used to get food at a certain time, but it will adjust to the new routine fairly quickly. If you are worried about your calorie intake, then you don't have to. In fact, most of the time we will keep our calorie intake the same when we start intermittent fasting because some people simply eat bigger meals to compensate. When we delve deeper into the book, you will realize that IF is one of the simplest strategies because it requires very little change in our behavior. That means IF is easy and simple enough so you can get on with it while being effective enough that it will make a difference.

In addition to the alternating eat-fast periods, there is one more rule. You cannot eat anything during the fasting period, but you can still drink water, coffee, tea, and other non-caloric beverages. That means you can still get your morning coffee fix before you head to work if you must. Some other forms of intermittent fasting also allow a small amount of low-calorie food during the fasting period, and we suggest you look into that further if it suits your fancy, although we do not recommend you sticking to those routines. If you need supplements, then they are allowed as well, so long as there are no calories in them.

While the idea of starving yourself for extended periods of time may seem ludicrous to you, it is actually a part of our evolution. Ancient hunter-gatherers did not have supermarkets to get food from, nor do they have refrigerators to preserve their food, nor do they have food year-round. They had to make do with that they have. As such, there were times when there was nothing to eat. So, humans evolved to be able to last long periods of time without food. In reality, fasting now and again is more natural for our body than eating 3 or more meals a day.

Fasting is also done for religious or spiritual reasons, such as Christianity, Judaism, and Buddhism.

The Effect of Intermittent Fasting

Intermittent fasting now combines the benefits of crash diet, therapeutic fasting, and alkaline fasting and avoids their disadvantages. As with the crash diet, the intermittent fasting also reduces the calorie intake, but this does not happen so excessively. The result is that metabolism does not radically shut down. So we get our energy consumption in our body, so we build an energy deficit. This deficit is compensated by the fact that will be burnt slowly.

The main drawback of the crash diet is the Yo-Yo effect. However, since we do not use intermittent fasting as a temporary, but as a permanent diet, this effect is exactly the same. We do not go back to an old diet, we keep it there, but in a reduced form. So our body simply does not get a chance to rebuild its fat.

Furthermore, the diet is unhealthy during a crash diet because it is very one-sided. However, when it is time to eat again, you can just as well provide what you want, and your body needs. The diet is healthy.

During the crash diet, you have a constant and strong hunger feeling. So you need a lot of discipline. However, when it is time to eat again, this feeling of hunger will soon disappear, and there are easy ways to deal with it. The chance of quitting the diet is thus low.

Therapeutic fasting has the advantage that the body can cleanse and regenerate. Even during intermittent fasting, the body is given the opportunity to cleanse and regenerate. Although the effect is not so strong within a short period of time, it is long lasting and achieves more over the years.

As therapeutic fasting, you will adapt with the intermittent fast to feel fresh and natural again. You will be able to distinguish between a simple appetite and true hunger. This means you can reduce the amount of food eaten.

Alkaline fasting flushes the acid out of the body. The intermittent fasting is able to do this, albeit slower. This simply happens because you continue to drink water and tea when you fast. Thanks to intermittent fasting, you do not need to eat new food, because you create a neutral environment in your body, which allows it to gradually dissolve the stored acid and excrete it through the urine.

You avoid the disadvantage of alkaline fasting that you spend more time shopping and in the kitchen. You do not need to buy or prepare any other food. You continue to prepare food and eat normally. However, since you eat fewer meals thanks to the fasting times, you also need less to shop and prepare.

What Should Be Considered

Intermittent fasting alternates a phase of eating with a phase of fasting. This has several advantages, which we have already mentioned in the previous chapters. But there are a few things you should keep in mind as well.

The positive success of the fasting depends very much on sufficient fluid intake. Let's be honest with ourselves, which one of us actually drinks enough? Probably none and that is up to us. We renounce the most important method of detoxifying our body because we have learned to always hold ourselves back. Shake off this false restraint once, and we can heal ourselves.

For drinking, it is best to drink water. Tea is good, too, but we should drink unsweetened tea. Coffee is also possible, but you should not overdo it, and if you drink it, please do it without sugar and milk.

In our body, the fluid provides several means for our well-being. First of all, our body can produce enough blood. Thin blood means better care for our organs and our skin. This also creates a better skin appearance, and it combats diseases and inflammation.

For drinking, the rule of thumb is that we need three liters a day. We drink two liters of it and take another liter over the food to us. That is not really enough. Why? Because we also want to detox right now and, ladies, we also have that time of the month. This fluid loss must also be compensated. This means that we should drink three to four liters a day and that adds to the water in the food. You do not have to worry about that, there is no such thing as too much drinking. If you actually take too many fluids, everything that's too much is simply eliminated. And, this is very important now, every time you go to the bathroom for the little business, you always say goodbye to some poison from your body. Therefore, drink a lot and let the poison disappear.

Now it is not easy for some women to break the habit. So, if you're actually struggling to drink enough, always pour something into a cup or a glass, and keep sipping it. This will soon become a habit, and you will feel much better.

For the food, you just continue to eat as before. However, you just need to do so a bit differently. You want a calorie deficit. Therefore, with meals, we eat exactly the same as before. Then, when you feel the first effects, you can make the meals smaller. They should not be much smaller, but always in small intervals.

Furthermore, you should make sure that you get enough energy. We know that one or two of you now want to lose weight very fast and combines intermittent fasting with dieting. This is fundamentally wrong. You want to feel good, and that means you need enough energy. So just eat normally when you eat and lose weight when you fast.

The food should be balanced over time. This does not mean to miss the beloved steak, the hamburger or the pizza, but to decorate it with enough other things. Then you also get all the things that your body needs, which means you get enough protein, minerals, trace elements, vitamins and whatever else. You do not need to make a big science out of it, just enough vegetables and something to eat from everything. Whenever you feel the desire to dine very healthily, then you just bring a fish on the plate. Fish contain just about all of the valuable nutrients our body needs.

Women should also listen to their bodies. We have a little bit more specific needs. This means that sometimes we have to bend the rules of the intermittent fasting a bit and sometimes fast for less than an hour. This is especially true during menopause. We should not forget only one important rule. We do not really change what we eat. In other words, we do not balance fasting by eating more during the mealtime. Then everything will be fine.

Fasting is very simple. You have an interval with food and an interval with fasting. As shown earlier, we would already be practicing it if we simply skip breakfast. You may be wondering if intermittent is that easy. Well, yes and no.

The stomach and the intestine must be empty so that the intermittent fasting actually produces beneficial health effects. This means that the time without food must be long enough for the stomach and intestine to process the last meal and then shut down. Only then does self-cleaning and healing begin.

The minimum amount of time that has to pass for fasting, i.e. the period without food, is 12 to 14 hours. That varies depending on the person. This results in various forms of intermittent fasting that you can choose for you individually. You should always listen to your body and also experiment a bit so that you can find exactly the form that suits you.

Overall, there are three common forms of intermittent fasting that are suitable for women. Because intermittent fasting mainly deals with when you should eat, meaning the hours, you can be flexible. The below methods are recommended for women but don't stick to them if it doesn't suit you. If you want, you can even create your own routine, so long as there is enough time for the body to clean itself. That means, your routine should have about 12 hours of fasting at least. Without further ado, let us look into some of the famous IF methods that many people use.

Chapter 4: Weight Loss and Health Goals

In this chapter, we will discuss planning your weight loss and health goals. You should write down what they are, both in short term and long term because these goals help you stay on track and make you feel accountable for yourself, which is also a motivational factor. Here, we will go over a 12-week protocol some say have been effective to build up their tolerance to fasting. This protocol is suitable for both newbies who have never fasted before, and veteran fasters alike. While you can follow this plan, you can always customize it to your preference, as your experience may vary even if you follow this plan to the letter. This guide is not tailored to any type of individual.

Week 1-2

Here, we will go on the time-restricted eating, also known as intermittent fasting. If you are new to fasting, we recommend you experiment with this first. We have previously discussed the 16/8 method, and while this is a common way people fast intermittently, you may find it tricky to get used to this.

So, you can ease your way into the 16/8 method by first fasting for only 12 hours and leave the other 12 hours to eat. Your eating phase could be between 7am to 7pm, 8am to 8pm, etc. You get the picture. Basically, you just need to pick any 12-hour window and eat within that time frame. So, if you eat your first bite at 7am, then you should try to consume all your calories before 7pm. That includes coffee and everything else. Then, you do not consume anything other than water between 7pm to 7am. Considering that you sleep for two-thirds of your fasting phase, the remaining four hours should be a breeze.

You should practice and master this for two weeks straight before you move on to the next step.

Week 3-4

After your body has adapted to the initial fasting cycle, the next step would be to ensure that you finish eating dinner at least three hours before bedtime. This is because we want the stomach to be empty so your body can relax, therefore optimizing your sleep and wake cycle. If you have food in your stomach by the time you are in bed, your body would still be active as it needs to digest the food, so you would feel restless. This is known as circadian rhythms.

Many people have had the experience of eating late, having wild dreams, and poor quality of sleep, not to mention waking up feeling like a bag of potato. To make matters worse, some may even experience acid reflux. Because we maintain our circadian rhythms because we are creatures of habit. These rhythms are the internal clock that tells us when should we sleep and when should we wake up. Before the clock was invented, we have already developed these rhythms and we sleep when it gets dark, and get up when it gets bright again. The clock in our brain is known as the suprachiasmatic nucleus that is sensitive to light, and it tells our body when is it time to go to sleep based on the light that comes through the retina. This clock coordinates with other body clocks such as one in the liver using neural or hormonal signals, core body temperatures, or eating and fasting cues.

That is why people always say that you should turn off your electronic device before you go to sleep, as they emit blue light that tells our body that it is still daytime, although it is already 1am. You may have the habit of snacking late at night or looking at your phone when you should be sleeping. Most of the time, you may find that you do not have a good sleep at all, as these activities throw off our internal clocks.

For instance, as the sky darkens, the clock in your brain detects the time change and signals to the body to prepare to sleep. However, you decide to eat dinner, probably a very hearty one. Then, your liver receives information that fuel is now at its highest as your body digests food instead of preparing to rest. Just like that, we are out of sync. Then, after dinner, you sit and watch TV or video on YouTube or browse social media on your electronic devices, which shower your eye with blue light that stimulates the clock in your brain, confusing it and making it thinks that it is still daytime, inhibiting the natural release of melatonin, which is a hormone that promotes and regulates sleep pattern. Maybe you skip watching TV and instead pour yourself a glass of wine or have some late-night snacks. This also creates circadian dissonance between the brain as it sees that it is dark outside, therefore time to sleep, and the body which is full of energy from the snack, the energy that it thinks you need to spend within the next few hours. So, when you eat at night, your brain tells the body to sleep, and the body responds by saying that this is not the time to sleep because there is energy to burn. This may be you, and you can easily see how you can mess your body up.

So, the key here is to sync your internal clocks, both in your brain and body, by stop eating after 7pm. Allowing your stomach to be emptied while you are upright will correct the mixed message you send between your brain and body. As a rule of thumb, you should stop eating anything 3 to 4 hours before bedtime so your stomach can empty itself completely before you sleep. If you haven't done this already, do this for 2 weeks straight before moving on. If you have been doing this since the start, you should still do this for another two weeks. It is imperative that you focus on synchronizing your circadian rhythms for these two weeks before moving on.

If you have problems keeping temptations at bay, you may need to make it harder for you to indulge in your cravings. For instance, instead of piling foods and snacks in your fridge, keep just enough food for a couple of days. If possible, get rid of all the treats you have around the house so you would not feel tempted. The visual sight of snacks might just be the cue your body needs to start craving, so get rid of them. Of course, there is no stopping you from going out late at night to buy a couples tubes of Pringles, but are you going to do that just for a snack? Most likely not. By making it very inconvenient for yourself to grab snacks, it is a lot easier for you to overcome temptations.

Week 5-6

Okay, so your body is now used to the 12 hours alternating fasting/feeding cycle and you allow your stomach to be emptied before bed. Good. Now, it is time to shrink down on your eating window. From this point on, you only have 8 to 9 hours of feeding time, with the remaining hours dedicated to fasting. This is the 16/8 method which we already covered, and should be practiced for 2 more weeks.

Week 7-11

Now, we are stepping things up to the OMAD or ESE method, also known as the 24-hour fast. When your body is starting to get used to fasting for 16 hours at a time, it is time to start fasting for 24 hours at a time, once a week. It can be breakfast to breakfast, lunch to lunch, or dinner to dinner. Of course, as your body is not adjusted, not to mention that you go on long hours without food, you can expect to feel very hungry, especially around the time you usually eat. When you do, it is important to remember that hunger comes and goes in waves, and they do not last longer than 10 minutes. So, if you manage to hold yourself together, or somehow distract yourself, you should be fine.

Start by fasting for 24 hours every 7 days. From there, you can try the 16/8 method every other day, and the ESE/OMAD method twice a week for the next three weeks. That way, you can build up your tolerance to longer fasting, which you should start in week 10. After you have done a month of 24-hour fasting, we recommend you try a 36-hour fast before moving on to the next step.

Week 12

Finally, it is time to take on the most difficult fasting challenge yet. Here, you will need to fast for 3 days or 72 hours. For more experienced fasters, you can even extend this to 4-5 day fast. As a general rule, it is not recommended that you practice a 3-day (or any longer) fasts more than once per quarter.

If you pair these fasting regimens with a clean diet, such as a plant-based ketogenic diet, you will lose weight, gain metabolic fitness, vitality, and longevity.

Other Tips

Before you start, there are a few things you can to do help you on this fasting regimen, especially towards the end.

First, and most importantly, you will feel hungry. This is very normal, and this is only temporary. Around the time when you usually eat, your stomach will start to grumble, and this is when you feel the hungriest. This is a normal part of the homeostasis to ensure that you are well-fed. This is how your body keeps things in balance. You will know when you start to crave when you start thinking about what you want to eat, or what you are in the mood for.

However, that can change. Researchers have found that humans can disrupt their own eating cycle after engaging in a 72-hour fast. Basically, after you have grown accustomed to fasting for 72 hours, you will not necessarily be hungry at the same times you were before you fast.

That means certain excuses will no longer be valid. Are you a night snacker? Do you always need something to chew on at 2pm? Well, this eating pattern can be disrupted. Your body is adaptable. All you need to do is to give it the tools to create better rhythms. You can do that by working your way up to the 72-hour fast.

This may surprise you, but the longer you fast, the less hungry you will get. This may go against common sense, but there are plenty of studies out there that support this fact. The benefits you will get from fasting far outweigh a grumbling stomach. Being hungry is nothing to worry about.

Chapter 5: Dieting

Just like exercising, fasting will only be effective only if you also control what you eat. You want to make sure that you eat healthy food that gives you enough calorie and making you feel full. In this chapter, we will discuss some of the food you want to include in your diet alongside your fasting plans so you can lose as much fat weight as possible without compromising your health.

Filling Food

You eat less if the food you eat makes you feel full faster, and what you eat determines how full you feel. Different food affects fullness differently. For instance, you feel full from eating boiled potatoes or oatmeal than from croissant and ice-cream for the same number of calorie. In order to feel full with the latter, you would need to consume an astounding amount, which also means consuming a ridiculous amount of calorie, which leads to weight gain. Filling foods can ward off hunger and help you eat less at the next meal. But what makes a food filling?

There is a term used to explain the feeling of fullness and loss of appetite after eating: satiety. To measure this effect, a scale known as the satiety index was created in 1995 in a study that tested 240-calorie servings of 38 different foods. On this scale, foods were ranked according to their ability to sate hunger. Foods with a score higher than 100 means that they are more filling, whereas foods scored under 100 are less filling. That means by eating food that scores more than 100 on the satiety index can help you eat fewer calories. Of course, when practicality is considered, no one wants to break out their calculator and satiety index chart. You can determine whether food is filling based on the following characteristics:

- Low in energy density: It means that the food is low in calories for its weight. Low energy density foods are very filling as they usually contain a lot of water and fiber and are low in fat.
- High in volume: It means that the food contains a lot of water or air. This might help increase their satiety score as well.
- High in fiber: Fiber provides bulk and helps you feel full for longer by slowing down the emptying of the stomach and increase digestion time.
- High in protein: According to some studies, protein is the most filling macronutrient, not to mention that it changes the levels of many satiety hormones such as ghrelin and GLP-1, allowing you to feel full faster and longer.
- As a rule of thumb, whole, unprocessed foods are usually more filling than processed foods.

As such, filling food should be incorporated into your diet plan so you can lose more weight in the long run. Here, we will look at 15 filling foods you should try out.

Boiled Potatoes

Potatoes are very nutritious, although they taste bland. Cooked, unpeeled potatoes are a good source of many minerals and vitamins, such as potassium and vitamin C (24345983). Because potatoes are high in water and carbs while containing moderate amounts of fiber and protein and almost no fat. Potatoes are very filling compared to many other high-carb foods.

In fact, boiled potatoes have a whopping high score of 323 on the satiety index, which put it on #1 of all 38 foods tested (7498104). Compared to croissants, which scored the lowest, potatoes score nearly 7 times higher.

A study found that eating boiled potatoes with pork steak result in lower calorie intake for the meal compared to combining it with white rice or pasta. A protein proteinase inhibitor 2 (PI2) which may suppress appetite is also found in potatoes, according to some evidence, making them more filling (2255726, 20820171).

Eggs

Eggs are very healthy and nutrient-dense. Most of the nutrients are in the yolks, which is where the chick draws its nutrients from as it develops and hatches. Antioxidants lutein and zeaxanthin, both of which may be beneficial to eye health (10426702), are found in the yolk as well. Eggs are a great source of protein. A large egg alone has 6 grams of protein, including all the 9 essential amino acids. Moreover, eggs also score high on the satiety index, meaning that they are very filling (7498104).

A study (16373948) found that eating eggs for breakfast instead of a bagel may increase your fullness and result in fewer calorie intake over the next 36 hours. Another study (23446906) also found that breakfast rich in protein, which includes eggs and lean beef, increase fullness and help people make better food choices.

Oatmeal

Oats, when eating as oatmeal (porridge) are also a popular choice for breakfast. Being low in calorie and a great source of fiber, especially beta-glucan which is a soluble fiber, and its ability to soak up water, give it the third place on the satiety index.

According to a study (26273900), participants reported feeling full and less hungry after eating oatmeal, compared to breakfast cereal. Subjects also ate fewer calories during lunch. Soluble fiber like the beta-glucan in oats, may make you feel full quicker and also cause your body to release satiety hormones and delay the emptying of the stomach (19753601, 19917449, 21115081).

Fish

Fish is also a great source of high-quality protein and rich in omega-3 fatty acids, which are essential fats that we need from food. According to a study, omega-3 fatty acids may increase the feeling of fullness in overweight or obese people (18602429). Moreover, other studies suggest that the protein found in fish may have a stronger effect on fullness compared to any other sources of protein (7498104).

On the satiety index, fish score the highest compared to any other protein-rich foods, including eggs and beef. Fish is ranked third out of the 38 foods tested. Another study also compared the protein found in fish, chicken, and beef. Researchers found that the protein found in fish has the most powerful effect on satiety (1542005).

Soups

While the evidence is mixed (14649371, 15639159), common sense dictates that liquids are often less filling than solid food. Soups, however, are a different story. Research (23818981, 23093339) shows that soups might be more filling than solid meals containing the same ingredients. In a study (23093339), volunteers consume a solid meal, a chunky soup, or a smooth soup that went through a food processor. From there, the feeling of fullness is measured as well as the rate of which the food left the stomach. Smooth soup had the biggest impact on fullness and is the slowest to leave the stomach, followed by the chunky soup.

Meat

Meat such as lean meats is also very filling according to reports on NCBI (20339363, 18282589). Beef scores 176 on the satiety index and it can have a very powerful effect on satiety. Beef is actually ranked right after fish in terms of protein content (7498104, 18689555). A study published in 1990 on NCBI (2228407) found that people who consume high-protein meat at lunch ate 12% less at dinner, compared to those who had a high-carb lunch.

Greek Yogurt

Compared to regular yogurt, Greek yogurt is very thick and rich in protein. As a breakfast, Greek yogurt is a great alternative to eggs. It is also a popular afternoon snack that might fill your stomach up until dinner, allowing you to eat less. According to a study published in 2013 on NCBI (23022602), which is conducted on women, subjects consume a 160-calorie yogurt snack that was low, moderate, or high in protein. Subjects who consumed high-protein Greek Yogurt feel full the longest, and ate dinner at a later time compared to women who consumed lower calorie yogurt.

Vegetables

Vegetables are also very nutritious as they are full of all sorts of vitamins, minerals, and many plant compounds that are beneficial for your health. They are rich in water content and low in calorie, containing fiber and fill you up very quickly. Of course, the only drawback is that they are not as delicious, but they take a whole to chew and are very satisfying. A study published in 2004 on NCBI (15389416) shows that a large salad before a meal of pasta increase the feeling of fullness and reduce the calorie intake for that meal.

Cottage Cheese

Cottage cheese is also low in fat and carbs, but dense in protein. As mentioned earlier, high protein food can help you feel full quicker, even when you consume a few calories. A study (25772196) found that the filling effect of cottage cheese is similar to that of eggs.

Legumes

Legumes, such as peas, lentils, peanuts, and beans, are also very nutritious. Loaded with fiber and plant-based protein but has a low energy density, legumes are very filling. An article (24820437) reviewed nine randomized trails that observe post-meal fullness using pulses which are a part of the legume family, found that subjects feel 31% more full compared to pasta and bread.

Fruit

Fruit also has a low energy density just like vegetables. They are rich in fiber, meaning that their digestion will be slow so you would feel full longer. On the satiety index, apples and oranges score very high at around 200 (7498104). However, we want to stress that eating whole fruits is different from drinking fruit juice. The latter is very unhealthy, and not very filling (19110020).

Quinoa

Another good source of protein is Quinoa. In fact, it has all the essential amino acids and they can be consumed as a complete protein source (18489119, 10719563), not to mention that is higher than most grains. Therefore, Quinoa is also a viable option to help you feel full and consume fewer calories.

Nuts

While we are on the subject of grains, nuts such as walnuts and almonds are also dense in energy and rich in nutrient. Their size allows them to be a perfectly healthy snack alternative to chips. Because they are high in healthy fats and proteins, they are also very filling. In fact, a study (19144727) shows that chewing almonds for only 40 times will greatly reduce your hunger and increase your feeling of fullness, compared to chewing for 10 or 25 times. So, have some almonds handy and start counting.

Coconut Oil

Coconut oil contains a special combination of fatty acids that are about 90% saturated. It consists mostly of medium-chain triglycerides and these fatty acids turn into ketone bodies when they enter the liver from the digestive tract. According to some studies (17228046), ketone bodies can reduce your appetite. Another study reported that individuals who eat breakfast with medium-chain triglycerides consume much fewer calories at lunch (9701177). Another study also looks at the effect of long-chain triglycerides and medium-chain triglycerides. According to the researchers, individuals who ate medium-chain triglycerides consume about 256 fewer calories a day.

Popcorn

Okay, let us get this out of the way. We do not mean the sweet popcorn you buy at the cinema. The healthy option here is the popcorn you prepare yourself in a pot or air-popper machine. A little bit of fat can increase the calorie content significantly.

Popcorn is a wholegrain food that is rich in fiber and 112 grams of popcorn has about 16 grams of fiber. Some studies discovered that popcorn is more filling than many other popular snacks such as potato chips or chocolates. So, if you cannot get almonds for some reason, popcorn is a healthy alternative. There are many things that make popcorn filling, including its high fiber content and low energy density.

Chapter 6: Women and Fasting

While the women's bodies function differently from men, that does not mean that they cannot enjoy the benefits of fasting. The only problem is that it is more difficult for women to maintain their fasting as they are expected to be hard at work for their families both at the workplace and at home. Sure, their husbands may have a higher income, but the entire family will crumble without women. There are children to feed, clothes to be washed, floors to be vacuumed, and food to be cooked. Women are expected to manage almost everything and excel at doing so. Frankly, it is outright impossible unless they have 48 hours a day to do everything. Alas, that is not the case, and we all live our lives in a constant rush, always under pressure and hardly have any time to relax. Women also have to deal with "that time of the month" that just makes their day all the more dreadful.

This section will cover some of the things that women need to know when they start fasting, particularly the complications they will face, how to deal with them, as well as other practical tips to make the entire experience more enjoyable for them.

Is it Suitable for Women?

Because intermittent fasting has become more and more popular in recent years, many people have many questions. Its popularity is thanks to the fact that intermittent fasting does not tell you what to eat, unlike most diets. It instead focuses more on when you should eat them by incorporating regular short-term fasts into your routine.

That way, you can consume fewer calories, lose weight, and lower your risk of diabetes, heart disease, and other diseases altogether, all within your own time. However, because the female body functions differently from that of the male, some studies have suggested that intermittent fasting may not be as beneficial for women. So, women need to use a modified approach in order to get the most out of their experience.

A study showed that blood sugar control actually worsened in women after they have fasted intermittently for three weeks, which was not the case for men. Some women have reported that they experience changes to their menstrual cycles after they have started intermittent fasting. This change is linked to the extreme sensitivity to calorie restriction in the female body. When calorie intake is low, a part of the brain called the hypothalamus is affected, which is the part that is responsible for hormone release.

Here, the lack of calorie intake disrupts the secretion of a hormone called gonadotropin, which helps release two reproductive hormones: luteinizing hormone and follicle stimulating hormone. Irregular periods, infertility, poor bone health, and other health effects result from the lack of communication between these two hormones and the ovaries.

While there are no comparable human studies, theses on rats have shown that alternate-day fasting over 3 to 6 months caused a reduction in ovary size and irregular reproductive cycles in female rats. As such, it is recommended that women should try out a modified approach to intermittent fastings, such as shorter fasting phase and fewer fasting days.

The Advantages of Fasting for Women

Fasting in our body combines the positive effects of crash diets, therapeutic fasting, and alkaline fasting, without carrying over their negative effects. If you must look closely, the only negative effect if intermittent fasting is that it takes some time to be effective. Still, the effects are there, and they are sustainable, not to mention natural and healthy for your body. In addition, intermittent fasting offers us a lot of benefits, especially for us women. Let's have a look at them in detail.

The Meals

Women, in particular, are affected by every kind of diet change, as it is still them who often work in the kitchen. So as soon as they want to eat something else or go on a diet, the burden of the change lies with them.

Intermittent fasting allows them to shop and prepare our food as usual. You like soups, well, eat your soups. You love fries, then bring them here. You fancy a decent steak; you do not have to slow down. Everything you eat so far, you continue to eat as usual. The conversion does not require you to start immediately reducing the amount of food you prepare. That comes with time by itself. So you cook everything as usual. But you can only miss a meal, but we'll get to that later. But that means you buy less and less often at the store.

A study found that young men ate up to 650 fewer calories a day when they only had 4 hours to eat for the day. Another study on 24 healthy men and women utilized a longer, 36-hour fast on eating habits. While subjects did consume extra calories after the fasting day, their total calories balance dropped by 1,900, which is a significant reduction.

A Better Sense of Well-Being

Intermittent fasting brings the poison out of the body, slowly and steadily. You will soon feel better and stronger. With that, you can do something again and enjoy life. Also, your organs work better, which actually gives you more power and allows you to do more.

Your Skin Gets Better

Here comes a real advantage for women. They just want a tight, healthy skin without wrinkles so they can look young. Intermittent fasting flushes the acid out of the body. The connective tissue becomes firmer and more flexible again. This tightens your skin and makes it shine, making it look much younger and wrinkles less.

The acid also often causes your skin to look unwell. So scales and lichens are often a consequence of the acid. This creates a welcome environment for fungi and bacteria, which then lead to an infection that leads to dandruff. Intermittent Fasting now allows the body to carry the acid out. The milieu on the skin changes. The natural protective film can regenerate. The fungi and bacteria will have a hard time settling down, especially when there is greater resistance. This means that the scales and lichens disappear. Likewise, you can say goodbye to eczema and pimple.

Your Nails and Hair Get Better

The acid also attacks the nails and hair. As soon as the acid leaves the body, they can regenerate. Your nails will be nice and shiny as your hair gains in volume and shine. Intermittent fasting thus acts like a total rejuvenation on your body.

The Fat on the Stomach Disappears

Intermittent fasting does not give the body enough energy. It has to feed on the fat and will attack it. Slowly and steadily you will break down your fat on your stomach and everywhere else in your body, where fat has accumulated. Do not expect a miracle. You will not lose 5 kilos a day or a week, but it is about one to three kilos a month. However, since this is done steadily and has a year of 12 months, you can easily figure out when you will have reached your desired weight.

Better Mood

Many women know that food dictates their mood. The food is supposed to give them energy, but all too often it puts pressure on their minds. It pollutes their body and thus their mind, but it also has a direct effect on our mood. Now, if you take a break by not eating, so you do not need to stress yourself about cooking, you'll soon feel lighter and happier again. Last but not least, intermittent fasting also relieves your digestion, giving you more energy. More energy means a better sense of well-being means a better mood.

A Better Sleep

Eating too much ensures that the body does not rest properly. The result is a restless sleep that lacks the important deep sleep phase. You cannot relax and do not feel rested. But with intermittent fasting, this is a thing of the past. Eating less means that your body can switch off more easily and get a deeper sleep. When well-rested, you are better equipped to take on the next day.

Heart Health

Heart disease is one of the leading causes of death worldwide. Leading risk factors for the development of heart disease include high blood pressure, high LDL cholesterol and high triglyceride concentrations. A study on 16 obese men and women showed that intermittent fasting lowered blood pressure by 6% in eight weeks, not to mention lowered LDL cholesterol by 25%, and triglycerides by 32%.

This is only one study, though. There is a lack of connection between intermittent fasting and the decrease of LDL cholesterol and triglyceride levels, there is a lack of consistency as to how much when the subjects are put through intermittent fasting. A study conducted on 40 normal-weight individuals found that during the four weeks of intermittent fasting during Ramadan did not result in a reduction in LDL cholesterol or triglycerides.

So, we need higher-quality studies with more robust methods before researchers can fully understand the effect of intermittent fasting on heart health.

Diabetes

Intermittent fasting may also be useful in managing and reducing your risk of developing diabetes. Just like continuous calorie restriction, intermittent fasting seems to reduce some of the risk factors of diabetes by lowering insulin levels and reducing insulin resistance.

In a randomized controlled study with more than 100 overweight or obese women and six months of intermittent fasting, it is reported that the insulin levels by 29%, and insulin resistance by 19%. Blood sugar levels,however, remained the same.

Another study conducted on pre-diabetic individuals over 8 to 12 weeks of intermittent fasting resulted in lowered insulin levels by 30% and blood sugar levels by 5%. In terms of blood sugar level, intermittent fasting may not be as beneficial for women compared to men.

A study found that blood sugar control actually worsened for women after 22 days of alternate-day fasting, while men experience no drawbacks. Despite this side effect, the reduction in insulin and insulin resistance would still reduce the risk of diabetes, especially for women with pre-diabetes.

Weight Loss

As we have explained earlier, intermittent fasting can be an effective and simple way to shed some weight over long periods of time, making it very sustainable. You can do it as regular short-term fasts as well and you will be able to shed a few pounds. Many studies suggest that intermittent fasting is as effective as calorie-restricted diets for short-term weight loss.

A 2018 review of studies on overweight adults found that intermittent fasting led to an average weight loss of 6.8kg over 3 to 12 months. Another review found that intermittent fasting reduced body weight by 3 to 8% in overweight or obese individuals over 3 to 24 weeks. Moreover, its participants reported that their waist circumference by 3 to 7% over the same amount of time.

It is also worth pointing out that the long-term effects of intermittent fasting for women remain to be seen. In the short term, though, intermittent fasting seems to help in losing weight. However, how much you lose will most likely depend on how many calories you consume when you are not fasting, and how long you follow this fasting lifestyle.

Other Health Benefits

A number of studies on animals and humans suggest that intermittent fasting may yield other health benefits such as:

- Preserve muscle mass: Intermittent fasting seems to be effective at retaining muscle mass, which helps you burn more calories even when you are resting.
- Increased longevity: Intermittent fasting has been shown to extend lifespan in mice and rats by 33 to 83%, but such an effect is not confirmed in humans.
- Improved psychological well-being: A study found that eight weeks of intermittent fasting decreased depression and binge eating while improving body image in obese individuals.
- Reduced inflammation: Some studies show that intermittent fasting can minimize key markers of inflammation, which is a big deal as chronic inflammation can lead to weight gain and many other health problems.

Best Types of Fasting for Women

There is no one-size-fits-all approach when it comes to dieting as many people may have different results even when they follow the same fasting regimen. Fasting is not an exception. As a rule of thumb, women should take it easy and follow a modified approach, as we have mentioned earlier. Shorter fasting periods, less frequent fasting or even consuming a small number of calories on the fasting days are recommended for women. Here are some variations of the fasting methods we have previously discussed:

- The 16/8 Method: Fasting for 16 hours a day, and eat all you need in 8 hours. Here, women are advised to start with 14-hour fasts and work their way up to 16 hours.

- Crescendo Method: You can fast between 12 to 16 hours twice or thrice a week. Fasting days should not be consecutive and they should be spaced evenly across the week.

- ESE/OMAD: To do this, you can start from 14-16 hours fast by following the 16/8 method first, and then work your way up to 24-hour fast. You should do this only once or twice a week.

- Alternate-day fasting: Here, you fast every other day but on your non-fasting days, you eat normally. For women, they can consume 20 to 25% of their usual calorie intake (roughly 500 calories) during fasting days.

- The 5:2 diet: Also known as the fast diet, you restrict your calorie intake to 25% (roughly 500 calories), and fast for two days a week, and eat normally the other five days. Allow one day between fasting days to allow the body to rest.

Whichever you choose, it is crucial that you eat well during non-fasting periods. So, healthy food is the way to go as eating unhealthy, calorie-dense food will only counteract the effect fasting has on your body. Whatever you do, it is best to consult your doctor before you start, and listen to your body. Only follow a fasting regimen that you can tolerate and sustain in the long-term that does not result in any negative health consequences.

Getting Started

So, where to start for women? It is simple. In fact, chances are that you have done many fasts before. A lot of people skip breakfast or dinner, therefore following one of the fasting regimens we have discussed above. So, just choose one of the fasting methods above and give it a go. It may be easier for you to start with the Crescendo method, then 16/8, then 5:2, then alternate-day fasting, then ESE/OMAD, as the difficulty scale nicely. Using the method from Chapter 4, we suggest that you follow each method for at least 2 weeks so your body has time to adjust, then work your way up.

However, you do not necessarily need to follow this plan. An alternative is to fast whenever it suits you. You can skip meals from time to time when you do not feel hungry, or when you do not have time to cook. At the end of the day, what matters is finding a method that works best for you and your lifestyle, not which fasting method you choose.

Safety and Side Effects

Generally, we do not recommend women following the original version of any fasting regimen as it can be too much for their bodies to handle and cause many health complications down the road.

That being said, some studies have reported that fasting may introduce certain side effects such as hunger, mood swings, lack of concentration, reduced energy, headaches, and bad breath on fasting days. There are plenty of stories out there of women who said that their menstrual cycle stopped while following an intermittent fasting diet, most likely a result from the lack of interaction of certain hormones with their ovaries, which we have mentioned previously. If you have a medical condition, you should also consult with your doctor before trying out intermittent fasting.

Women should consult doctors if they:

- Have fertility problems or a history of amenorrhea (missed periods)
- Are pregnant, breastfeeding, or trying to conceive
- Are underweight, malnourished, or have nutritional deficiencies
- Have diabetes, or regularly experience low blood sugar levels
- Have a history of eating disorders

As we mentioned time and again, your mileage may vary when you fast. Most of the time, you will do just fine. However, if you ever notice or experience any problems, such as loss of your menstrual cycle, you must stop immediately.

Chapter 7: Autophagy

You may have tried juice cleanses and detox diets, and they are just bluffing to get you to buy their products using pseudoscience. Of course, there is nothing wrong with drinking your weight in liquid kale, but it does not clean your body any faster than actual food. The key here is to actually understand how your body cleanses itself. Thankfully, it is a process that you can control. All you need to do is practice a little self-cannibalism. Okay, it does not involve you chomping down your arm.

The practice of training your body to eat itself is something you should strive forward. This is a natural process known as autophagy, literally meaning self-eating. It is the body's system of cleaning house. Basically, your cells create membranes that seek out scraps of dead, diseased, or worn-out cells, devour them, break them up for parts and use whatever usable to create energy or new cells. It's your body of recycling old, weak, and useless cells to create better, healthier ones. Recycling is good, right?

According to Colin Champ, M.D., a board-certified radiation oncologist, assistant professor at the University of Pittsburgh Medical Center, and author of Misguided Medicine, autophagy allows us to be more efficient with the resources in our body by getting rid of faulty parts, stop cancerous growth, and halt metabolic dysfunctions such as diabetes and obesity.

There is also evidence suggesting that autophagy also has a role in controlling inflammation and immunity. When scientists engineer rats that are incapable of autophagy, they are lazier, slow, and are more susceptible to high cholesterol and impaired brains. Autophagy is, therefore, the key to slowing the aging process by allowing your body to swap out dysfunctional parts and replacing them with better ones to allow it to function better. You can learn how to trigger the process of reconstructing your body.

3 Ways to Autophagy

"So, how do I eat myself?" is probably the sort of question you could not even imagine asking yourself. There is one thing you need to know here are all the three methods follow the same formula. You see, autophagy is a response to stress. So, the idea here is to put stress on your body to kickstart the auto-cannibalism mechanism into gear. Of course, no one likes stress, but short-term discomfort now will bring about long-term benefits. So, how do you stress yourself out?

Exercise

We all know how unpleasant it can be to be sweating bullets, making all that embarrassing grunts, and going through the post-workout pains. But here's the thing: exercise stresses your body. Actually, in order to allow your muscles to grow, you need to damage it. That is the entire point of working out. When you cause tiny microscopic tears on the muscles, your body rushes to heal those wounds, ending up making your muscles stronger and more resilient against any further damage you might put them through.

A lot of people do not realize that regular exercise is the most common way that they use to cleanse their body. That is why you feel fresh and energetic after working out. `

A study in which scientists engineered mice to have glowing green autophagosomes, which are the structures that form around the pieces of cells your body wants to recycle, found that the mice have greater cell recycling rate after they ran for half an hour on a treadmill compared to when they are in a relaxed state. The rate was still going up when the mice ran for 80 minutes. Here's the fun thing about it: the result was so surprising and inspiring that the lead scientists decided to buy a treadmill.

But of course, the study was conducted on mice. What about humans. We are different from rodents, after all. Daniel Klionsky, Ph.D., a cellular biologist at the University of Michigan, specializing in autophagy said that it is difficult to determine the level of exercise we need to stimulate autophagy and the extent to which the process is upregulated. However, it is already clear that exercise has many benefits other than stimulating autophagy, so it is already a good idea from the start. If you love pushing yourself by doing tougher exercises, then it is even better. Colin Champ recommends relatively intense exercises if you want to reap maximum benefits.

Fast

We have talked about this extensively, but fasting also stresses the body. If you have been drinking juice to cleanse your body, then now is a good time to stop because it actually works against autophagy. Skipping meals is something that you would not feel pleasant about, but will benefit from in the long run.

In fact, research has shown that there are many benefits from fasting, even when you only do it occasionally. We have discussed some of them in a previous chapter already, two of which are lowered risks of diabetes and heart disease, both of which might be linked to autophagy.

There is also research on how fasting promotes autophagy in the brain, which means that it could be a way to lower the risk of neurodegenerative diseases such as Parkinson's or Alzheimer's. Other studies have also shown that intermittent fasting improves cognitive function, brain structure, and neuroplasticity, meaning that you can learn easier. However, it is not clear if autophagy was the cause. Moreover, the studies were conducted on rodents, and we cannot assume the benefits will be the same for us.

Lower Your Carb Intake

As mentioned previously, there are many ways to fast. Some people fast 18 hours a day a few times a week. That may be too much for beginners. A study published on 11 February 2011 on the multiple roles of autophagy in cancer showed that it is possible to have a lower risk of heart disease if you only fast for one day a month. Forgoing food occasionally seems to work, but there are other ways to get similar benefits without giving up eating comfort food.

This is called ketosis, and it is also an incredibly popular diet regime among bodybuilders and anyone who wants to have better longevity. The idea is to cut down on carbohydrates to a level so low that the body has no other alternative but to burn up the body fat to fuel itself. Therefore, ketosis is a good way to lose body fat without affecting the muscle. There is some evidence suggesting that ketosis helps the body fight cancerous tumors, lower the risk of diabetes, and protects it against brain disorders, especially epilepsy. Moreover, another research found that more than half of children suffering from epilepsy have at least a 50% reduction in seizures after going on the diet.

Colin Champ said that Ketosis is like an autophagy hack. You can trigger the same metabolic changes and benefits from fasting without actually fasting. It is worth noting that keto diets are high in fat. About 60 to 70 percent of your calories should come from fat. That means lots of steak, bacon, and peanut butter shakes. Protein only makes up about 20 to 30 percent, and carbs are always below 50 grams a day.

However, if you find that staying in ketosis is harder than not eating altogether, there is an alternative. Similar benefits have been found in people following a diet with carbs not exceeding 30 percent of their overall calories.

Other Alternatives

Unfortunately, there are not. However, you can bet that there are incentives for researchers to trigger autophagy from the use of pills. Of course, we all want to look for ways to trigger autophagy through chemicals, and you may find claims on the internet through a quick Google search. After all, taking pills is a lot easier than putting yourself on a diet. However, we are a long way off from having reliable chemicals, so we suggest that you avoid it altogether.

We mentioned previously that ketosis was observed to have reduced epileptic seizures in half in children. There are also anti-epileptic drugs that are being developed that produce the same effects of ketosis. Should its development is successful and it is made available to the general public, it is possible that those pills are the key to trigger autophagy with no effort at all.

However, you should not get your hopes up. There are just so many metabolic changes that happen during ketosis. So, mimicking all of them with a pill might be outright impossible. It may be necessary to put your body through all of the stress that comes with ketosis to get all the benefits.

Still, there is absolutely no need to torture yourself by fasting extensively, or staying in ketosis for an extended period of time, or exercise intensely all day every day to gain all of those benefits. Only a few hours of any of the above is enough to get autophagy going.

Chapter 8: Other Practical Tips and Guides

In this chapter, we will discuss other tips you can incorporate into your fasting regimen to optimize your weight loss.

Other Weight Loss Tips

While fasting and intermittent fasting will put you on a good path toward weight loss, there are a few more things you can do to shed a few more kilos without compromising your health, energy, or mood. As you may already know, there is plenty of buzz surrounding weight loss, and you may have heard some ridiculous things that people do to lose weight, especially when there is no science backing it up. Over the years, however, scientists are finding new ways to get rid of weight effectively and healthily. Here are some of them.

Water

People often say that drinking water help with weight loss, and that is true. Drinking water boosts metabolism by 24 to 30% over 1 to 1.5 hours, allowing you to burn a few more calories. In addition to drinking water frequently, you can also drink water before meals, as a study showed that drinking only half a liter of water about half an hour before meals help dieters consume fewer calories and lose about 45% more weight, compared to those who don't.

Eggs for Breakfast

Whole eggs have many health benefits, including weight loss. Studies show that when you replace a grain-based breakfast with eggs, it helps you eat fewer calories for the next 36 hours in addition to losing more weight and body fat. If you do not eat eggs, that is fine. You can get the same effect by consuming any high-protein food for breakfast.

Coffee

Have you ever noticed that, after drinking coffee, your hunger seems to just fade away? Coffee has been demonized unfairly. In fact, quality coffee is full of antioxidants and can have many health benefits. Many studies have sown that the caffeine in coffee can boost metabolism by 3 to 11% and increasefat burning rate by up to 10 to 29%.

It is recommended that you drink black coffee as it is low in calorie. Also, make sure you do not add sugar or other high-calorie ingredients to your coffee. That will just negate any benefits.

Green Tea

Just like coffee, green tea has many health benefits, one of which is weight loss. While it has a small amount of caffeine, it is full of powerful antioxidants called catechins, which works with caffeine to enhance fat burning. While scientific evidence is mixed, many studies agree that green tea can help you lose weight all the same.

Glucomannan Supplement

Many studies have shown that a fiber called glucomannan is linked to weight loss. Glucomannan absorbs water and sits in your gut for a bit. Think of it like a sponge. While it is in there, you feel more full and thus make you eat fewer calories. That way, you can lose a bit more weight.

Added Sugar

Added sugar is probably one of the worst things to have in a modern diet. A lot of people consume way too much of this stuff. Numerous studies have shown that the consumption of sugar and high-fructose corn syrup is associated with an increased risk of obesity, and other conditions such as heart disease and type 2 diabetes. If you want to lose weight, cut back on added sugar. Of course, it is easier said than done. Before you buy anything, make sure to read the labels because even some "health foods" can be chock-full of sugar.

Sugary Drinks

While we are on the subject of sugar, avoid sugary drinks such as soda and fruit juice. Sugar alone is bad enough, but sugar in its liquid form is even worse. Some studies show that calories from liquid sugar might be the leading cause of fat increase in the modern diet. For instance, a study shows that sugar-sweetened beverages are linked to a 60% increased risk of obesity in children for each daily serving. Here, it is worth mentioning that this also applies to fruit juice as well. While it tastes like fruit, it actually contains almost the same amount of sugar as any other soft drink like Coke.

So, if you want something sweet in your mouth, eat whole fruit instead as it's a lot healthier. If you can't, then at least try to minimize the number of sugary drinks you drink.

Refined Carbs

Similarly to added sugar, you should also avoid refined carbs like the plague because refined carbohydrates have sugar and grains that have been stripped of their nutritious, fibrous arts. This includes white bread and pasta.

Studies have shown that refined carbs can cause a major spike in blood sugar, leading to hunger, cravings, and increased food intake a few hours later. Many cases of obesity are linked to the consumption of refined carbs. If you do wish to consume carbs, make sure to eat them with their natural fiber.

Low-Carb Diet

If you wish to get all the benefits of carb restriction, perhaps you should go all the way and commit to a low-carb diet. Many studies have shown that such a regimen can help you shed twice or even thrice as much weight as a standard low-fat diet while also improving your health.

Smaller Plates

Sometimes, you can trick your brain into thinking that you eat the same amount of food when you are actually eating less by using smaller plates. You may be used to portion your food based on how it fills your plate, so this trick may work for you. This has been shown to help some people eat fewer calories without realizing it. However, this does not affect everyone. The most noticeable effect is when this is done on overweight individuals.

Portion Control or Calories Counting

Portion control, or basically eating less, or counting calories can be very useful for obvious reasons. Some studies have shown that keeping a food diary or taking pictures of your meals can help you lose weight.

In fact, anything that increases your awareness of what you are eating is most likely to be beneficial.

Healthy Food Around

Instead of having snacks like chips laying around the home, tempting you every time you step into the room, why not replace them with healthy food? That way, when you become excessively hungry, you can snack on some healthy food instead. Your choice of snacks should be easily portable, and simple to prepare such as whole fruits, nuts, baby carrots, yogurt, and hard-boiled eggs.

Probiotic Supplements

Taking probiotic supplements that have bacteria of the Lactobacillus subfamily has been found to reduce fat mass in our body. However, this only applies to the lactobacillus subfamily, not the entire lactobacillus species. Some studies suggest that L. acidophilus actually causes weight gain.

Spicy Foods

Another trick you can use is by eating spicy food. For example, chili peppers contain capsaicin, which is a spicy compound that boosts metabolism and reduces your appetite slightly. However, that does not mean that you can lose a lot of weight just by eating spicy food over time because you may develop tolerance to the effect of capsaicin over time, which might limit its long-term effectiveness.

Aerobic Exercise

Another excellent way to burn calories and improve your physical and mental health is by doing aerobic exercise. It seems to be effective for losing belly fat, as the unhealthy fat tends to build up around your organs and cause metabolic disease.

Lift Weights

One of the worse side effects of dieting is that it often causes cause muscle loss and slow down metabolism, which reduces its effectiveness in terms of reducing fat weight. This slowdown and muscle are otherwise known as starvation mode.

One way to prevent this is by doing some resistance exercise such as lifting weights. Some studies have shown that lifting weights can help maintain a high level of metabolism and prevent you from losing muscle mass.

Of course, losing fat does not necessarily result in a toned body. You should also build up your muscles through resistance exercise.

Fiber

Fiber is often recommended for weight loss, although the evidence is mixed about this matter. Some studies show that fiber, especially viscous fiber, can increase satiety and help you control your weight for a long time.

Vegetables and Fruits

It should go without saying that eating vegetables and fruits is a lot healthier than fries and pizza. Vegetables and fruits have many properties that make them effective for weight loss because they contain a lot of fiber, but very few calories. They also have high water content, which means they have low energy density but also very filling. As such, they prove to be very effective for weight loss, not to mention that they are very nutritious.

Chew Slower

It will take a while for your brain to register when you have eaten enough. If you eat quickly, then you would have already been overeating for quite a few bites already before your brain tells you that you had enough. Some studies show that chewing slower help you consume fewer calories and increase the production of hormones linked to weight loss. Moreover, you should also chew more thoroughly as they may reduce the calorie intake at a meal.

Sleep

Sleep is very underrated, and it may be the key to weight loss. Studies show that poor sleep is one of the biggest risk factors for obesity because it is linked to an 89% increased risk of obesity in children and 55% in adults.

Overcome Your Food Addiction

A recent study conducted on Americans and Europeans found that roughly 20% of them fulfill the criteria for food addiction. If you have food cravings and cannot seem to cut down on your eating no matter how hard you try, you may be a victim of food addiction. If that is you, then you should seek professional help as trying to lose weight without first overcoming food addiction is nigh impossible.

Protein

Protein is one of the most important constants in your weight loss equation. Having a diet mainly comprised of protein has been shown to boost metabolism by 80 to 100 calories a day while cutting off roughly 440 calories a day off your diet. A study shows that by having protein as a source of 25% of your total calorie intake reduce obsessive thoughts about food by 60% while also reducing the desire for late-night snacking in half. So, adding protein into your diet is a clever way to lose weight.

Supplement with Plant Based Protein

While we are on the subject of protein, if you have problems getting it into your diet, consider taking a supplement, such as protein powder. A study shows that replacing some of your calories with Plant based protein can cause weight loss of about 8 pounds over time while also increasing your muscle mass.

Whole, Single-Ingredient Foods

More commonly known as real food, you can become leaner and healthier if you do yourself a favor and eat whole, single-ingredient foods. They are filling by nature, so it is very hard to gain weight if you base your diet on them.

Eat Healthily

Sometimes, diets may not work in the long term for you. We have already established that the same diet plan will have different effects on different people. Some studies show that dieting may lead to future weight gain. Instead of following a diet regimen, maybe you should just eat healthily. Aim to become healthier, happier, and fitter. It may be more effective for you to focus on nourishing your body instead of depriving it. Weight loss should come to you naturally then.

Common Mistakes when Fasting

Fasting is not that new anymore, yet only a few really know about it. As a result, many people often get it wrong. This results in unsuccessful, unhealthy fasting, which would raise criticism against fasting as a whole. To prevent this, let's talk about the 5 biggest mistakes so that they can be avoided from the outset.

The first and most important mistake is not to overthink fasting as a whole. For intermittent fasting, all you need to do most of the time is skip breakfast. You only eat lunch and dinner, and you're good to go. That's all there is to it. Also, if you do decide to dig further into the matter, make sure you consult your doctor and do thorough research. The last thing you want to do to your body is something that you do not really know about. As mentioned earlier, you may overeat. This is often aggravated by the idea that you fast (and yes, the ones covered in this book are proven to be successful). But after fasting, you do not eat reasonably. You eat a lot more than you should just to compensate for the loss of calorie during the fast. This is because let's say you skip breakfast to fast, you become hungrier. When lunch times come around, you eat a lot more.

Together, this means one thing. You would not reach the calorie deficit, and may instead build up a surplus in your body, causing it to become even fatter. So, if you want to get into fasting, do your due diligence and research thoroughly so you know what you want. As mentioned previously, consult your doctor before you attempt to fast because you may have certain medical technicality that prevents you from doing so, or make the experience a living hell. Moreover, you should have a general plan that includes a general idea of the nutritional value of food. Of course, you do not need to take out your calculator and start counting calorie. But you should know a few things like pizza contains enough energy you need for the whole day and that a hamburger has multiple times the calories of a salad.

If you want to get it right, you need a plan and this plan must start from your current state, which is the time before you start fasting. What calorie quantity and nutrient distribution was there at that time? From there, you need to look at your calories intake, how much you want and how do you want this to be distributed over the day. How much meat, how much fries, how many vegetables, and so on.

Another mistake that people often make is that, whether they have a plan or not, when they start fasting and finish their first fasting phase, they develop cravings. This often happens, but people often lose control when there are temptations right around the corner. They eat too much and they lose their progress. Intermittent fasting, for example, does not mean alternating between fasting and feasting. It means that fasting is followed by a meal phase, which is the time when you feed yourself normally before fasting again. Of course, the initial phase of food deprivation will lead to craving, but you need to do everything in your power to resist.

Intermittent fasting is a diet that requires minimal willpower and perseverance compared to a crash diet or a compete fasting diet. We mentioned this plenty of times previously, but we want to stress that intermittent fasting requires absolutely no effort or will. You just need to be in control in the beginning. It helps to know that you will get to eat again very soon. However, just because it requires no effort does not mean that you can lower your guard. You need to maintain your fast during the fasting phase, and the subsequent fasting phases for this to work. Because fasting does not yield an immediate result, it may be disheartening to see that you have made little progress over the week. As mentioned earlier, fasting is a sustainable method of weight loss. You can just stick to your usual diet and fast to start losing weight.

There are two things that are helpful. The first is the plan which we mentioned earlier. It is something that you can stick to. It does not help if you plan out everything and then ignore it. You absolutely have to follow this plan. The second thing that helps is the knowledge that cravings will eventually pass. Once you have gone through some fasting phases, your body will get used to it and it just does not ask for more. Then you will be perfectly comfortable with your 8 hours daily fasting and no longer feel that cravings.

However, those who indulge in their cravings, do not just cancel the effect of the intermittent fasting immediately. It aggravates theirsituation because the cravings lead to too many calories being consumed, which deposit themselves as fat, but also too many unhealthy foods will be consumed to satisfy their taste buds. This introducestoxins into the body and further damaging the body and reduce its performance. You really have to work the first few days on yourself and make sure that you eat normally after fasting.

The third mistake is just the opposite of the second mistake, which is the lack of food. This usually happens because you want to force results, instead of being patient and achieve a lasting effect. The body will respond by switching to starvation mode. This means it lowers metabolism rate to preserve energy. As a result, you do not have enough food for yourself and at the same time, you still do not lose weight. This can lead you into a vicious cycle, because you may reduce your food consumption even further so you may lose more weight. But then you will soon feel like in a crash diet. It is no longer comfortable and the body will start feeding on your muscles. If then the nutrition is given too low, threatens the yo-yo effect, where it will store even more energy the next time you eat. Until then, however, you will feel limp, has no energy and is prone to depression.

The fourth mistake is the excessive supply of coffee. Unfortunately, coffee drinking is still allowed during intermittent fasting. There's nothing wrong with that, as long as the coffee is drunk in moderation. At the same time, coffee has a satisfying effect. This then leads to more and more coffee, so you do not feel hungry. The effect is devastating. Coffee is not the problem and it actually inhibits the appetite, which makes you fasting, especially in the morning, good. But if a cup is not enough for you, then the whole thing will be different. It gets really problematic when you drink up to three or four cups.

When you drink coffee during your fast, it gets into the blood much faster and much more. The result is the release of adrenaline and cortisone. Both of them have an appetite-suppressing effect because these are the hormones that are supposed to make it possible to escape or fight, and hunger is an obstacle. At the same time, both hormones bring energy to the body. But they break up the sugar in the blood and the body gets the power that it needs for the fight or the escape. But the blood sugar level drops and what stays behind when the effect of the hormones has stopped is a craving for sweets. This then makes the fast even more difficult or ensures that sugar will be consumed in a large quantity for the next feeding phase.

The fifth mistake is the wrong organization and the wrong execution of meals. So the body or the digestive system should start slowly after fasting first. It is recommended to eat something easy for the body, such as at breakfast. Most people, however, just skip breakfast but then eat something heavy for lunch. This then burdens the digestive system, which now consumes a lot of energy to break down the heavy food. That also means that we have much less energy for our other tasks. We are then tired and tired and cannot get up to anything. It is better, even at noon, to start with something easy to tolerate, instead of overburdening our stomach and overwhelming ourselves with it.

The sixth mistake is to approach the matter too rigidly. It makes sense to have a plan, but it cannot anticipate or factor in all uncertainties. Here, you have to be flexible and able to react to the circumstances. So, for example, if you have to go on a business trip, are invited to an important party, or the daily routine is otherwise disrupted, you have to be able to react and adjust your planning. The important thing is that the exceptions really remain exceptions and the changes are not a habit.

Common Weight Loss Mistakes

Losing weight can be tough for many people. Sometimes, you feel that you have followed everything to a T, and yet you still do not get the results you were promised. When that happens, it is easy to become frustrated because you put yourself through everything but only getting little to no results. If that is you, maybe you have made one of these common mistakes:

Focusing on the Scale Weight

It is very common to feel that you are not losing nearly enough weight despite the fact that you do your very best to follow a diet regimen. However, the number of the scale does not tell the whole story. It does not mean that you are still fat. The scale is not the only way to measure weight change. Weight is actually comprised of many things such as fluid fluctuations and how much food is still in your system. Moreover, there is also muscle mass to consider if you exercise regularly. The point of fasting and weight loss isn't about weight specifically, but rather the fat weight in your body. In fact, your weight can fluctuate by about two kilos over the course of the day, depending on how much you eat and drink.

Things are even more complicated for women. You see, certain hormonal changes in women such as the increase in estrogen levels can lead to greater water retention, which also prevents them from losing weight.

In any case, there are many factors that make the scale spit the same number at you. What matters here is not what the scale says. You may already be losing fat weight in your body, which is a great thing. Sometimes, the number does not change simply because your body retains water. Thankfully, you can do many things to lose water weight.

Moreover, if you have been working out, the muscle mass you accumulate throughout the workout routine may even outweigh the fat loss, which might give you the illusion that the fast or any diet regimen you have done is ineffective. A good way to tell if you are losing fat weight is when you put on your clothes. You may feel that they are looser, especially around the waist, even though you have a stable scale weight. Your waist circumference may go down, and you can measure that by using a tape measure, or take monthly pictures of yourself so you can compare how much fitter you have become since you have started.

Too Many or Too Few Calories

To any extreme is detrimental, and this also applies to fasting and weight loss. While a calorie deficit is needed to lose weight, it can be counterproductive as they can trigger the body's emergency starvation mode which slows down metabolism and may lead to muscle loss. Slower metabolism rate means your body spends less energy, meaning that you will have a calorie surplus next time you eat, which will lead to weight gain, not to mention that you may feel horrible. Studies show that very low-calorie diets less than 1,000 calories a day can lead to muscle loss and slow down metabolism significantly (19198647).

For several years, it is believed that if you have a daily calorie intake any lower than 3,500 a week would result in about 0.5kg of fat loss. However, more recent studies show that calorie deficit varies from person to person, so a baseline cannot be established here. You might feel that you are not eating as many calories, but the reality is that we all tend to underestimate and underreport how much we eat.

According to a two-week study on ten obese people (1454084), subjects reported to consumed only 1,000 calories a day and the subsequent lab testing showed that they actually took in in about 2,000 calories a day. There are a few reasons why we underestimate the number of calories we eat, one of which is that we eat healthy food that is high in calories such as nuts and cheese. The key to controlling how much you eat is by watching your portion size.

Too Little or Too Much Exercising

It is natural to be losing muscle mass as well as fat mass during weight loss, although how much you lose them depends on many factors. If you do not exercise at all while fasting, you may lose more muscle mass and experience a decrease in your metabolic rate.

On the other hand, exercising might also help you minimize how much muscle mass you would lose while maximizing fat loss and prevent your metabolism from slowing down. The more lean mass you have, the easier it is for you to lose and continue to lose weight.

However, as we have mentioned previously, to any extreme can be detrimental. Over-exercising is a problem as well. Some studies show that excessive exercise is not sustainable for many people in the long term, and may lead to stress (23404767, 26707388, 23667795).

Moreover, it may even impair the production of a hormone that regulates stress response called adrenal hormones. It is neither effective or healthy to force your body to burn more calories through excessive exercising.

Instead of lifting excessively, feeling sore and drained at the end of your session so you can force your body to burn those extra calories, you should instead take it easy and lift weight or do cardio several times a week instead. That way, you establish a system of sustainable weight loss and maintain a relatively high metabolic rate.

Not Lifting Weights

While we are on the subject of exercising, you may not lose weight because you are not lifting weights enough. Lifting is a form of resistance training and is very important for weight loss. A large number of studies show that lifting weight is one of the most effective ways to gain muscle and boost metabolic rate, in addition to improving overall body composition and boosting belly fat loss.

In fact, there was a review of 15 studies with over 700 people and they found that the best way to lose weight seems to be a combination of weightlifting and aerobic exercise (24358230).

Low-Fat or "Diet" Foods

Natural, whole foods are considered to be some of the healthiest things you can put into your digestive system. Because there is a growing health craze about weight loss, many companies exploit this need and put out processed low-fat foods or "diet" foods, which may not be as good as they sound. They are actually loaded with sugar so they taste better.

For example, a cup of low-fat, fruit-flavored yogurt has up to 47 grams of sugar, which is roughly 20% of the yogurt. Instead of keeping you full, these "low fat" products will make you hungrier and you might even end up eating more as if eating that much sugar in such a small amount of food is not bad enough. So, instead of eating those foods, eat only the foods that are not processed, nor as minimally processed as possible in combination with other nutritious foods.

Overestimate Calorie Burned During Workout

A lot of people believe that exercise puts their metabolism on overdrive. It is only partially true at best because exercises increase the metabolic rate slightly, but it is actually very underwhelming. Studies show that both normal and obese people often overestimate how much calories they burn during exercise, often by a large amount. Another study had participants burn between 200 and 300 calories during exercise sessions. Subjects reported that they had burned more than 800 calories, and this led them to believe that they can eat more, which they did (21178922). That being said, we do not mean that exercising is useless for weight loss. It is still important for overall health and it can help you shed a few kilos. The problem is that it is not as very effective at burning calories as you may think.

Not Enough Protein

If you want to lose weight, getting enough protein is critical to your success. In fact, protein has been shown to help people lose weight in many ways. It can reduce your appetite, increase your feelings of fullness, increase your metabolic rate, decrease your calorie intake, and help protect your muscle mass during weight loss.

According to a 12-day study, participants ate a diet with 30% of its calories coming from protein and they consumed on average about 575 fewer calories a day compared to a diet with 15% of its calorie coming from protein (23221572). Another review found that higher-protein diets that contain 0.6 to 0.8 grams of protein per pound may benefit appetite control and body composition (25926512).

So, you should consider optimizing your weight loss by making sure that your diet is rich in protein.

Not Enough Fiber

A low-fiber diet might also hamper your weight loss effort as well. Some studies show that viscous fiber, which is a type of soluble fiber, help reduce appetite by forming a gel that holds water. That way, the fiber moves slowly through your digestive tract, making you feel full longer because your stomach cannot empty them as quickly.

Research also suggests that all types of fiber benefit weight loss, not just viscous fiber alone. However, a review of many studies found that viscous fiber is the best when it comes to reducing appetite and calorie intake compared to other types of fiber (21676152).

When your total fiber intake is high, some of the calories in the food in mixed meals are not absorbed. According to some researchers, doubling your daily fiber intake can result in up to 130 fewer calories being absorbed into your body, meaning that you can increase the fiber content in your meal and you may absorb fewer calories although you eat the same amount of food (9109608).

Too Much Fat on Low-Carb Diet

Ketogenic diet and low-carb diet is not for everyone, although they can prove to be very effective for weight loss. Studies show that those kinds of diets can reduce appetite, which results in lower calorie intake. However, many low-carb or ketogenic diet allows unlimited amounts of fat, if the resulting appetite suppression can keep calories low enough for effective weight loss.

The problem is that people may not know when to stop eating when they are on this diet because their body does not receive a strong enough signal because the food is not very filling. So, by the time they feel full, they may already be consuming too many calories to reach a calorie deficit.

If your food or beverage has a lot of fat and you are not losing weight, consider cutting back on the fat and see how it works.

Frequent Eating

For many years, we have been told to eat every few hours to prevent hunger and a dip in metabolism. The issue here is that this can lead to many calories being consumed without actually feeling full, which can lead to overeating very quickly.

In a study, it is found that men who consume 3 meals within 36 hours experience a decrease in blood sugar levels and hunger while having a relatively high metabolic rate and feelings of fullness compared to men who eat 14 times over the same period of time (22719910).

There is also a misconception about the suggestion that you should eat breakfast every morning, regardless of appetite. According to a study, people who skip breakfast consume more calories at lunch compared to when they'd eaten breakfast. However, throughout the day, they consumed roughly 400 fewer calories (23672851).

This is where the eating pattern known as intuitive eating comes in because your body will tell you when it is hungry. Eating when and only when you are hungry seems to be the key to successful weight loss. However, that does not mean that you should let yourself get too hungry. It is better to have some snacks than to become starving, which can lead you to make poor food choices.

Setting Unrealistic Expectations

We understand that you should have weight loss and other health-related goals to keep you motivated, however you should ensure that you set realistic goals. Having unrealistic expectations can work against you.

Researchers went over a huge amount of data from many weight loss center programs and they reported that overweight and obese women tend to drop out of a program after 6 to 12 months, although they expected to lose the most weight (16339128).

So, when you design your own weight loss goals, do make sure that your expectations are adjusted to a more realistic and modest goal. If anything, it is better to set a low bar first and work your way up from there. It is a lot more motivating to see that you have achieved more than you initially expected, even if it is a modest goal than to see that you come short on your ambitious goal. A 10% drop in weight in one year is realistic, and such a goal can prevent you from getting discouraged and improve your chances of success.

Not Tracking Your Food

Another common mistake you may make during your fasting endeavor is the fact that you may be eating more calories than you need to lose weight. Eating nutritious food is a viable weight loss strategy, but this alone will not be enough.

If you do not know the nutrition value of the food you eat, you may not be getting the right amount of protein, fiber, carbs, and fat to optimize your weight loss. Some studies show that tracking what you eat can give you a clearer picture of your calorie and nutrient consumption, not to mention providing accountability (18617080).

In addition to food, many online tracking sites, and mobile application also allow you to put in your daily exercise to calculate your total calorie intake.

Tips to Stay Motivated

No diet and no fasting is really easy and even intermittent fasting needs willpower. However, there are ways to make the beginning easier and once the beginning is done, the rest is much easier. Therefore, we have summarized a few tips here, so you can easily start the new diet.

For instance, it is very easy to get started with intermittent fasting using the 16/8 method. Still, it may still be a bit hard for one or the other to not eat for 16 hours at all. In this case, one should approach the implementation of the fast slowly. The beginning is a change in the diet from fast food and mostly heavy dishes to light and healthy dishes.

A healthy diet, especially at the beginning, should not have bread, with the exception of wholemeal bread. You should be introducing healthy food into your diet after every fasting period. So you can still eat your usual food within the meal times, but during the fasting, you may eat salad or raw food. As a result, the body gets used to it so slowly that it is not constantly supplied with heavy food. This makes it much easier to get used to the real fast later on. At the start, you just set a meal that is the easiest for you. After a few weeks or months, you transition to another kind of meal. Then the next and in the end, you eat only lightly. Then you can start with the right fasting phase in the next step.

The fasting phase can be kept as-is at the beginning. As always, you can have your breakfast, lunch, snack, and dinner, which has now been converted to healthy stuff. Then, in the next step, you start to bring your dinner forward or, alternatively, to move the breakfast backward. No matter if you have decided on dinner or breakfast, you only move it by half an hour in one step. After a while, you approach it with another meal.

Those who have decided to have dinner will soon reach the time when there is no longer enough time between afternoon snack and dinner. Then it's time to merge the two together, creating a meal time to replace the snack time altogether. If you decided to have breakfast, it will eventually reach the point when it is too close to lunchtime. Then you cancel the breakfast and move the lunch a bit by moving lunchtime back slowly in 30-minute increments until it overlaps breakfast time and then shifts it to its original time.

Moreover, you can make the beginning of fasting easier by preparing mentally for it. It is important to know that pessimism is not a motivation. So if you accept starvation as motivation, there is no motivation to be found. You will, therefore, have no willpower to endure this. So, if you decided on trying out intermittent fasting, you need to have at least one important reason. Some people try it out because they are overweight, have health problems, or for any other reason. You need to know about this. The more you know, the more meaning it has and the more it motivates you. Then you can also withstand the hunger phases and avoid a relapse.

At the same time, you always have to bring positive thoughts. You should not think about hunger, but about the health, you improve. One should not say that one is weak without food, but the body has time to regenerate and to be stronger.

The 16/8 method is easiest for the body and the easiest to integrate into your daily routine. Therefore, you should actually work with your diet and slowly transition into this regime. Especially as a beginner, the 16-hour fast seems to be very long, but here's the thing: you can skip half of it by sleeping for eight hours. You do not eat anything while your sleep anyway, so you are already making big progress when you sleep.

Furthermore, you should not make a big deal out of fasting. It is mainly about the time of sleep. For the meal times, you move them around only a bit to better suit your schedule. The whole thing is so simple and therefore require neither great effort nor does it pose an insurmountable obstacle. So you are not putting yourself through a lot to get results.

When using the 16/8 method, you should not expect too much in a short time. Intermittent fasting and especially the 16/8 method aim at a slow and sustained weight loss. So if you try the scales, you will quickly notice that you only lose one to two kilos per month. But that's no problem because weight loss is progressing steadily without any implications.

If you also exercise while fasting, you may even gain weight under certain circumstances. This is because muscle cells are a lot heavier than fat cells. So, if you build muscles while losing fat simultaneously, you may either see little changes in weight or you may even gain weight. There is no need to be disheartened about this. The goal is to eliminate the fat in your body, which does not necessarily mean losing weight.Of course, it is important to see the progress in order to be motivated. But now we have just realized that you do not lose weight fast and, as you exercise, may even put on more weight. So how should you measure your success?

Success comes in two identifiable ways. The first is that you feel better and lighter. The body is not so much burdened by the toxins and regenerates over time. Accordingly, you feel energetic, fresh, and healthy. The second way also does not require a scale. You may not see your progress when you step on the scale and see your numbers, but you can feel the difference when you tighten your belt, put on your trousers, shirts, or when you buy new clothes, you may feel that you fit into them a lot easier. This is also more important than the kilos because after all, you do not want to lose them to be lighter, but to be slimmer, and that can be achieved very easily.

Fasting as a Lifestyle

Intermittent fasting is not just a diet. You can do it consistently, and above all, for a long time. Then you will not only be slimmer, but you will stay that way. Therefore, you do not just feel better for a moment, you feel better for a very long time. You can achieve a consistent result if you stick to these pointers.

Start Slowly

Intermittent fasting is not a diet. It's not for a short time, and it's not just about a few pounds. It's about continuing your normal diet over time, as usual, while slowly and steadily losing weight and improving your health.

Start intermittent fasting slowly and get used to it. Do not just forgo meals in the name of getting thinner. If you have trouble, we suggest you move two meals slowly together until they become one and then move that time to a meal time that works best for you.

You do not always have to adhere strictly to your eating time. If you have an appointment or a meeting, you can break out of your rhythm and plan another time to start fasting. Still, you should not constantly change the rhythms. Your body needs to adjust, and if you keep changing, it is the same as not having a consistent sleeping pattern. You will have your meal or enough sleep, but you will feel horrible every time.

Take Your Time

Do not expect and, most importantly, do not force rapid weight loss. This is not a sprint, and again, intermittent fasting is not a fast diet. The whole thing is a marathon. It's about a steady, slow weight loss. This is also much healthier for the body.

By the way, if you are doing sports at the same time, you may not even see any change in weight. That's because you build muscle cells and they are much heavier than fat cells. If you want to see your success, look at your clothes. You might notice that they are looser than before.

Never exaggerate

We have talked about a few intermittent fasting methods; the ESE method is one of the harder variants out there. We have also mentioned that you should experiment and find out which pattern works best for you. However, by "working best for you", we do not mean the method that yields the best result for you. The worst thing you can do to your body is overextending, trying to force a result, which is unsustainable and would often damage your health instead. Listen to your body. Try one of the three methods we discussed. Stick to a routine only if your body feels okay with. Do not force anything, because you'll only be frustrated and you'll destroy your motivation in the end.

Sleep

In the beginning, intermittent fasting is difficult. It is therefore important to always combine it with sleep as it will only bring you the slightest hunger. So you can then get started and from there and don't have to spend too much time going on an empty stomach.

Keeping Busy

Especially at the beginning, you think more about food than you should. This is normal among beginners. It was torture. There is a workaround, though. You can try focusing your energy on something else. That can be work that you should be doing, a romantic movie that you want to watch or a lovely date with your partner. Do what you like so you will not notice that you are hungry. Oh, and if you go to the movies or go out with a partner, leave the eating activity out of the plan.

Sports

Sport is a nice help, but not a must. However, if you can, you should invest your new time and money in a little physical exercise. With it, you build some muscles, and you also increase your performance. You also tighten your body and look better and younger. In addition, sport makes sure that you can reduce your daily stress and find better sleep. We will discuss sports and intermittent fasting in details in a later chapter.

Drinks enough and the right one

If you make intermittent fasting a part of your lifestyle, be sure to combine it with enough drinking. Detoxification does not work if you do not absorb water. In addition, enough fluid intake also prevents other ailments and illnesses. Basically, water is the simplest, cheapest and most effective medicine. Do not waste this opportunity for you and your body.

Find like-minded people

A hobby, occupation or lifestyle is much more interesting if you can share it with someone. Turn to the internet. Find forums and exchange ideas. Convince your partner and your friends. What you do together is twice as fun. In addition, the people around you also have great ideas, and it is fun to try them out together. After all, it is also the social interaction that gives us people the greatest sense of happiness and the lack thereof is often the feeling of dissatisfaction, which is at the beginning of too much food and overweight. So be in touch, and you will be pretty, slim, young, and happy.

Fasting and Sports

Intermittent fasting and fasting is a diet that is very easy to combine with sports. This will bring even better results. However, it also comes with its own problems. For that, you should also know which sport and how and when you should operate it.

Why Sports?

Our body is still in a time when it expects to face hardships. It expects to be challenged and be threatened. The reality is that we have never been any safer. We are very comfortable, and there is no need to spend a lot of physical strength to sustain ourselves. Because of that, our body keeps accumulating energy it expects to be used one day, which never comes. As a result, we put on a little bit of weight every day. That is why exercising is important. As soon as this happens, we will live much healthier and feel better.

Without exercise, the body, the muscles specifically, is not used or strained. Over time, your muscles will be weak, and you will eventually rue the day that you skip the exercise. Now, even if we don't exercise, our muscles will still be strong enough to allow us to walk around and do our tasks because we at least have trained them that much. That may be enough in most situations, but that's about all. What is the result? As soon as we push ourselves a little bit more, it will be too much. Worse still, when we spend a third of the day at work and come home, we feel tired and beaten and can do nothing more. The muscles will only be capable enough to do just enough work that you need to be done for the day. Do we really want that? For me, not really. Of course, we, especially women, need to do more than the bare minimum to get anywhere in life. That means cooking a delicious meal for the weekend, get that report done before the deadline, or attend a party. For that, my body should be able to handle a little more stress sometimes.

If we do not do sports, then we do not consume the stress hormones that we build up over the day. This means our body cannot rest completely and we cannot relax.

If we do not do sports, the body hardly sees a difference between day and night. This is because we spend most of the day depleting the mental energy, and not physical energy. So, even though we are mentally tired, the body is still quite energetic. This means we can hardly rest and get enough sleep and, above all, the quality of our sleep is not as great either.

Sport is so important in our lives. We make our bodies stronger so that we are better prepared for challenges and also for everyday life. Sport makes sure that we reduce stress and sport makes us sleep better.

Intermittent fasting helps us to detoxify our body. Sport, together with intermittent fasting, improves our health considerably. This is not least due to the fact that sport gets our circulation going, which is conducive to detoxification.

Sport together with intermittent fasting accelerates weight loss. But we do not just lose the kilos faster, we replace them with muscles and, while the scale does not show that, you will look better.

Speaking of better forms, the sport is also a means for correct aesthetics. We just look better, because the right muscles in the right places also bring out our shape better. At the same time, our skin becomes firmer and our wrinkles less visible.

What you also need to know is that muscle cells always burn fat, even when they are not in use when we exercise. This means that those who train for an hour a day to build muscle will lose weight 24 hours a day.

What Kind of Sport?

Just like intermittent fasting, you will need to find the one that works for you. Of course, the main idea here is to help you lose weight, not pack bulky muscles. So, lifting weight is out of the question unless you want to build muscles. If you are young, a whole-body workout is probably the best for you. If you are old, you should go for everyday sports.

A total body workout consists of various endurance and muscle exercises. The goal is to build the muscles evenly throughout the body. Do not worry, ladies, you will not become powerful men. We are not talking about lifting very heavy weights and extreme forms of training. We speak of some weights for the right muscle groups, and already the legs, hips,and stomach are well-formed and firm. Even the bosom will thank you. Just try it.

Everyday sport should also combine endurance and muscle training in itself. But there are different variants, ranging from very easy to difficult. Let's start with the simple part. If you are not so young, you should go for a walk. This brings a lot of fresh air into the lungs, and the whole body moves. At the same time, it builds a little muscle, but not too much that you have to worry. The most important thing here is to get the circulation going and strengthen it.

If you are young, you can do the walk at a brisk pace and a weight of one or two kilos in each hand. This will also get the circulation going and get a bigger impact on the muscles. If you are in the early stage of adolescence or really young, try going for a walk by jogging with the dumbbells in your hand. You get to actively work all of your muscles and consume a lot of calories. Above all, we will pump so much oxygen through our bodies that we feel young and fresh even hours after the exercise.

Another option is cycling. You can still engage all the muscles in your body this way. The circulation gets going as we pedal. This also trains our leg muscles, while holding the wheel also requires our other muscles.

The best option, however, is swimming. Here the circulation and every single muscle in the body is stressed. At the same time, the joints are spared from the strain. This will make everyone fast and slim, without fear of damage.

What Should a Training Session Look Like?

A training session consists of the warm-up, the actual training, and the transition phase. It's easy for everyday training. In the beginning, we go swimming or driving the bike a bit slower. This accelerates our breathing and our heart rhythm so that our body is prepared for the actual stress. This phase should be between 10 to 15 minutes long.

The next phase is the actual training. Here we run, swim and ride the bike in our real training pace. Here we should be careful to choose a pace at which we are still comfortable. We should not feel dizzy or hyperventilate. This phase lasts about 30 minutes.

The cooldown phase is the conclusion and should slow down the body. While doing this, you should feel your breathing slowing down. This phase should have the same length as the warm-up, i.e. 10 to 15 minutes.

The whole body workout works with weights. Here we should do jogging or biking as a warmup or cooldown, before and after we start using the dumbbells.

The dumbbell training takes place in passes. Each set consists of 10 to 15 repetitions (reps) with the same dumbbell and the same movement without stopping. We have to see for ourselves which weight is right for us. If we can do more than 15 repetitions in one go, we need to increase the weight. If we only make less than 10, then we have to use a lighter weight.

Each exercise should consist of 4 to 6 sets. Between the sets, there is a little break of one to two minutes. After each exercise, there is a break of 3 to 5 minutes.

Timing

It is also important to do sport at the right time and to ensure that it is properly timed throughout the week. Lighter everyday sports in the form of walking can be completed every day. All other sports need a firmer training regime.

During exercise, we damage our muscles. This is actually normal. Muscle growth is only possible by causing tissue damages to the muscles and growth comes when they start healing. This injury is the goal of the sport. Then our body repairs the damage and makes the muscles stronger so that next time they can stand more and do more. Nevertheless, we must keep this damage in mind and deal with it.

The first consequence of the injury is that we cannot exercise every day. There must be at least one rest day between training days so that the muscles have time to regenerate. This allows us to work a maximum of three days a week, with one day of training alternating with one day's rest.

Also important is the right amount of training time. Here, a distinction should be made between the 16/8 and ESE method. For the 16/8 method, sports should be done so that the end of the workout coincides with the end of fasting. This has two advantages.

First, we have no fresh food in our body. This means that throughout our training, our body uses its fat reserves to meet its energy needs.

Second, after training, our body needs a lot of building materials to regenerate. But since our fasting has just ended with training, we can now feed these materials through the food.

The Effect in Our Body

Training in our body provides a boost for the formation of muscles. By doing so, we force the body not to use his muscles to cover his energy needs during fasting. So it will, whether the body likes it or not, use up the fat reserves instead. This brings the maximum effect for our body in terms of looking better by exercising and losing weight by fasting.

Chapter 9: Conclusion

That is all you need to know to gain that beautifully toned body through fasting. Thank you for reading this far and we hope that you learned some valuable fasting tips.

Fasting is natural for your body, although the idea of intentionally depriving it of food may seem alien to some. The main reason why fasting works so well is the fact that we listen to our body and understand how it works. There are many ways to fast, each with their own strengths and drawbacks.

Whatever fasting methods you follow through, we suggest that you do so in moderation. Fasting is not a sprint, but a marathon. So, you want to make sure that you can stick to it for as long as possible. Listen to your body and stop when you feel that something is wrong.

Moreover, just like exercising, fasting only works if you control what you eat after. By following our guidelines, you should be well on your way to create a meal plan that is healthy, and nutritious without too much calorie to counteract the effects of fasting.

That said, we wish you luck on your weight loss endeavor and stay fit.

Intermittent Fasting Mastery:

The Practical Guide to Effortless Weight Loss and Healing your body for Men and Women With Autophagy, 16:8 Fasting, 5:2 Fasting and One Meal a Day (OMAD) and More

Contents

Chapter 1: Introduction

You may have heard of intermittent fasting. It is the current health and fitness trend, and for very good reasons. A lot of people talk about it and many questions have been raised. Some say that it allows them to lose weight over long periods. Others say that the idea is ludicrous. As far as we know, a lot of people use it to lose weight, improve their health, all within their own convenience. Many scientific studies have shown that intermittent fasting can have powerful effects on both your brain and body, not to mention that it may even improve your longevity. In this book, we will look into all the science behind intermittent fasting, how it works, all the common methods, which ones are for you, and much more about intermittent fasting. Without further a do, let us get into it.

What is Intermittent Fasting?

Intermittent, or IF for short, is more of an eating pattern than a diet because it involves an alternating cycle of fasting and eating. You just schedule your meals so that you can get the most out of them. That's it. You do not need to change what you eat to practice intermittent fasting, although it can maximize its effectiveness (more on that in a later chapter). What is important is when you eat.

Many studies show that intermittent fasting can help you lose weight, improve your metabolic health, improve your longevity, and strengthen your immune system. We will look into the science behind intermittent fasting and how it could combat obesity later.

Since IF is an alternative eat-fast pattern, there are many approaches to IF and the most notable difference among them is when you should and should not eat. The great thing about IF is that it is a great way to get slimmer without going on a crazy diet you saw on the internet or cut your daily calorie down to almost zero, making you feel miserable all the time. We all want a simple regimen we could stick to, and there is nothing simpler than intermittent fasting. Of course, while intermittent fasting is the easiest to follow, you will not see the results immediately. It takes time, but at least your weight loss is sustainable. You will get all the health benefits without torturing yourself in the process.

There are two main methods of fasting. The 16:8 is the most common form of fasting which involves 16 hours of fasting and 8 hours of eating period. The other one is calledOne Meal a Day method in which you fast for 24 hours at a time, only twice a week. There are other variations as well, and we will get to them.

Looking at the 16:8 method, you may be thinking that you have done some form of fasting already. That is correct. Does the term "break one's fast" sound familiar? That's what the word breakfast comes from. You break your fast which lasted for the whole duration when you were sleeping. If you sleep for 8 hours a day (and we hope you do) then you have been fasting for 8 hours a day already. Looking at the 16:8 method, we can easily achieve that duration just by skipping breakfast. If you eat dinner at 8 pm, then you just need to eat again at 12 am, considering it as your brunch. You'd already be fasting for 16 hours when you skip breakfast! See how simple it is?

Now, if you are unfamiliar with intermittent fasting, you might think that it is unnatural and unhealthy. After all, how can skipping meals be healthy? It does sound counterintuitive, but all diets all involve moving more and eating less. For IF, it is enough to just eat less. It is easier than you think, and many people have reported that they feel better and have more energy after fasting. Skipping a meal and resulting in hunger is not a problem either. While you may feel uncomfortable in the first few days of fasting, your body will adjust to the new routine quickly. The idea of IF is to lower your calorie intake to achieve a weight loss effect, but not too much so that it slows down your metabolism and your body starts using up your muscle mass instead of your fat mass. Later in the book, you will realize that intermittent fasting is one of the simplest strategies because it requires little change in our daily behavior. IF is simple and easy enough so you can implement it seamlessly into your life whilst being effective enough for it to make a difference.

Moreover, there is one more rule to the alternating eat-fast periods. Most fasting regimens strictly prohibit eating anything during the fasting period, however, you can still drink water, coffee, tea, and any other beverages that have virtually zero calories. That way, you can get your morning caffeine fix before you head to work if you want. Other forms of IF, especially modified ones, may allow a small amount of low-calorie food during the fasting period. These modified methods work the best for women and beginners alike as they can help you ease your way into fasting. However, you should go into full fasting mode whenever you can to achieve maximum effect. Supplements are also allowed as long as there are no calories in them.

Whilst the idea of starving yourself for an extended period of time seems crazy, you would be surprised to know that it is actually more natural for our body to starve once in a while rather than being fed thrice or more a day. You see, ancient hunter-gathers did not have supermarkets to get food from, nor did they have refrigeration or other preservative methods to make their food last longer, nor did they have food year-round. They had to make do with that they had. Because fruits and vegetables are not filling, and animals were not easy to hunt down, feasting times that were full of food were often followed by long periods of starvation. Our ancestors were used to eating so much at a time and then lasting through a long time of scarcity. We have evolved since then to last long periods of time without food. Our body was trained to stock up on as much energy as possible to spend when those periods of scarcity arose. Whilst scarcity is no longer an issue, our biological evolution takes its sweet time to evolve. Until then, fasting now and again is more natural for our body than eating three or more meals a day. Fasting is also done for religious or spiritual reasons, such as Christianity, Judaism, and Buddhism.

The Effect of Intermittent Fasting

IF combines the benefits of crash diet, therapeutic fasting, and alkaline fasting, whilst managing to avoid their disadvantages. With the crash diet, intermittent fasting reduces calorie intake without being too excessive about it. This results in a stable metabolism rate, meaning that we still use roughly the same amount of energy in our body. The lower calorie intake and stable energy consumption leads to an energy deficit, which means we lose weight.

The problem with the crash diet is the yoyo effect. Here, you will be hungry constantly, and it can be unbearable at times. For crash diets to be effective, you need a lot of discipline and a high level of willpower. If you give in to temptation, the effect can be drastic as you may eat a lot more than you should, gaining more weight to the point that it is even worse than the starting point. IF is a more permanent diet solution. Although the yoyo effect is there, the hunger is not as strong since you do not deprive yourself of calories that much. You can keep the old diet, but just make sure that you do not go overboard with the calorie intake so your body has the chance to replenish its lost fat. Because you keep eating whatever you used to eat, and fasting is not as intense, intermittent fasting is a lot easier to stick to.

Therapeutic fasting has its ups and downs as well. IF helps you feel fresh and natural again, so you can distinguish between a simple appetite and real hunger. This means you can reduce the amount of food eaten to keep your calorie intake relatively low.

Alkaline fasting works by flushing the acid out of the body. IF can achieve this as well, although it is not as fast. The acid level is reduced in our body as we drink water and tea when you fast. Thanks to IF, there is no need to change your diet since you create a neutral environment in your body that allows it to dissolve the acid and excrete it through the urine. Another thing that makes IF better than alkaline fasting is that you save yourself some time. For alkaline fasting, you need to spend time shopping and cooking. As mentioned previously in IF, there is no need to do that. You eat and cook as usual. The only difference is that you eat fewer meals as you need to fast. You also get more time for yourself, not to mention that you have more money to spend on yourself as well as you no longer need to shop as often.

What You Should Consider

IF is an alternating phase of eating and fasting. This form of eating has many benefits as we have previously discussed. However, there are certain things you should keep in mind as well.

IF works if you have sufficient fluid intake. Let's be honest with ourselves here. Do you actually drink enough water every day? Probably not. If this applies to you, then you should know that you are missing out on the most important method of detoxifying our body.

Start drinking plenty of water so your body has enough fluids to refresh the body once again. Drink water whenever you are thirsty because you are already dehydrated when that happens. If you just got out of bed, drink a glass of water before you do anything else. Your body has been deprived of water for about eight hours (assuming you sleep eight hours a day, and you should), you need a lot of water at the start of the day. Throughout the day, you can drink tea, but the unsweetened one is best. Whilst coffee is allowed, drink it sparingly and without sugar or milk.

Fluid has many benefits for our health. First of all, our body can maintain a good level of blood concentration. Thin blood means better care for our organs and our skin. This also gives us better-looking skin, whilst also allowing your body to combat diseases and inflammation.

As a rule of thumb, you need to drink three liters a day on average. Two liters we get directly from water, and one liter from the food we eat. Sometimes, three liters a day is not enough because we want to detox our bodies. For ladies, you also know that there is that time of the month when you lose a lot of bodily fluid. Such loss must be compensated. That means that you should drink up to four liters a day, and the extra liters compensate for the food if you are practicing IF. Drinking four liters may seem like an overkill, but it is nothing to be worried about, you need to be drinking a lot more water to put yourself at risk of overhydrating. Your body will get rid of the excess fluid. This is important because every time you go to the bathroom your body flushes out the toxins from your body. Therefore, drink a lot and often, so your body can get rid of the toxins in your body.

Some people may have a bad habit of not drinking very often and would end up feeling horrible from the dehydration. So, if you are struggling to drink enough water, try to have a glass of water full nearby at all times. Keep taking a sip as often as you can and it will eventually become a habit. You should start to feel better then.

As for the food, we will go more extensively into it in a later chapter, but you can just continue to eat as before. However, you just need to alter it a bit. You want to create a calorie deficit. Therefore, we eat as before only during specific eating window before cutting down on the calorie intake. There is no need to cut down on 500 calories a day, work your way down in intervals.

Moreover, you should make sure that you get enough energy. We understand that you want to lose weight very quickly by combining intermittent fasting with dieting. This is fundamentally wrong. You want to feel good, and that means you need enough energy to sustain yourself. So just eat normally when you eat, you will lose weight when you fast.

The food should be balanced over time. This does not mean to miss the beloved steak, the hamburger or the pizza, but you should complement them with enough other things. Then, you get all the things that your body needs, which means you get enough protein, minerals, vitamins, etc. It isn't rocket science. You just need enough vegetables and other things to satisfy your nutrition needs. Whenever you feel the desire to dine very healthily, then you can just include fish. Fish contains just about all of the valuable nutrients our body needs.

Women should also listen to their bodies as they have a little bit more specific needs. This means that sometimes they cannot follow the exact fasting regimen for reasons we will also talk about later. This means they need to follow a modified version that is both friendly for newcomers and women alike. In short, the effect of intermittent fasting can be really nasty for menopause. Again, there is only one rule to intermittent fasting. You skip a meal (or two... or three) and eat normally without trying to compensate for the meals lost.

Fasting is very straightforward. You have an interval with food and an interval with fasting. As shown earlier, we would already be practicing it if we simply skip breakfast. You may be wondering if intermittent is actually that easy. The answer is, yes and no.

The stomach and the intestine must be empty so that intermittent fasting actually produces beneficial health effects. This means that the time without food must be long enough for the stomach and intestine to process the last meal and then shut down. Only then does self-cleaning and healing begin.

The minimum amount of time that has to pass for fasting, i.e. the period without food, is 12 to 14 hours. That varies depending on the person. This results in various forms of intermittent fasting that you can choose for yourself individually. You should always listen to your body and also experiment a bit so that you can find exactly the form that suits you.

Overall, there are three common forms of intermittent fasting regimen. Because intermittent fasting mainly deals with when you should eat, meaning the hours, you can be flexible. If you want, you can even create your own routine, so long as there is enough time for the body to clean itself. That means, your routine should have about 12 hours of fasting at least. Without further ado, let us look into some of the famous IF methods that many people use.

Chapter 2: Problem with Obesity

Obesity has become so commonplace in America that one out of three Americans is obese. The American Association of Clinical Endocrinologists, the National Institutes of Health, and many other organizations now consider obesity a chronic disease. In fact, obesity is so widespread that it is considered to be a national epidemic in America, according to the Centers for Disease Control and Prevention. Obesity is not just a problem of weight alone. It may also lead to some more serious effects on a person's physical, metabolic, and psychological health. The problem is not solely on self-control.

To put it simply, your daily meals are just like your bank account. Your income is the calorie intake, which you would spend on physical activities throughout the day. When you take in more calories than you can burn, you have an energy surplus. Of course, having a financial surplus is a good thing, but you do not want to have too much energy surplus. This is oversimplified, as the situation is more than a matter of addition and subtractions. There are many other factors in play that make some people gain weight faster than others. So, how are we gaining weight?

Weight Gain Causes

There are seven common causes that lead to weight gain in many people. These include changes in our society and how we eat, all of which contribute to the increase in obesity.

Eating Differently

You may not notice it, but we all eat differently daily. On average, up to 60% of adults drink at least one sugary drink a day. Again, this is not only a matter of self-control. In America, food higher in sugar, salt, and fat are more widely available. There are fast food chains everywhere, offering high-calorie, unhealthy food at very low prices. The same can also be said for food vending machines and cafeterias in school. As such, it tends to cost more to eat healthily. Moreover, some people, especially those living in lower-income, minority, and rural areas often do not have access to stores that stock healthy, affordable foods such as fruits and vegetables. Portion sizes are often larger as well, especially for less-healthy foods and beverages.

Physical Inactivity

Let's face it. Not many of us get enough physical activity as we should. Depending on where you live, recreational centers and park may be very far away, not to mention that safe walking or biking routes may be limited. As such, cars have become the main commuting solution for many people. Other than that, students tend to not get enough physical education. In our homes, many chores are already mechanized as many tools are created to replace manual labor.

Couch Potatoes

Many Americans spend too much time in front of a screen, whether it is a TV screen or a computer monitor. We already work eight hours a day, and then we come home to spend more time staring at a screen. Children are not spared from this problem as children between the age of 8 and 18 years spend up to 7.5 hours each day engaged in entertainment media such as TV, computers, cell phones, movies, and especially video games. Roughly 4.5 out of 7.5 hours are spent watching TV.

This passive entertainment comes at a steep price. Not only that people would be detracted from other physical activity, but they also tend to have snacks and drinks whilst watching TV. The common image is of a person with a bag of chips and a can of coke, sitting snug on the couch watching TV. Moreover, watching TV exposes people to the advertisement of other high-calorie, unhealthy food, further reinforcing the habit of eating junk food.

Early Stoppage of Breastfeeding

Breastfeeding helps protect children from becoming obese. Unfortunately, out of 75% of mothers who breastfeed, only 13% of infants rely on just breast milk alone after six months.

Heredity, Diseases, and Medication

Of course, genetic conditions also play a role in the speed of which you gain weight. Genetic conditions such as Prader-Willi syndrome are a direct cause of obesity. Other genes and behaviors have been confirmed by scientists to trigger obesity. The genetic makeup of some people may make them more susceptible to obesity. Still, other factors are required to complete the picture.

Moreover, certain disorders such as Cushing's disease and hypothyroidism can also cause people to gain weight. On the flip side, some drugs such as steroids, antidepressants, and diabetes medication may cause weight gain as well.

To Sum Up

Overall, because of our behavior, socioeconomic status, culture, and environmental factors, we have gained much more weight than we anticipated. Moreover, hormones in our body can influence our metabolism. Eating habits also lead to weight gain.

As you can see, depending on where you live, it may be near impossible to lose weight. This is especially true in America as there are fast food outlets literally everywhere. It is not easy to resist temptation when the food we try to avoid is available at every corner. Whilst we cannot control what is on TV or what these fast food outlets sell, we can control ourselves. This is what intermittent fasting is all about – self-control.

What you need is not a short-term calorie restriction that makes you feel miserable. You need something that is a lot more sustainable. You want a dieting regimen that allows you to be flexible with your time, convenient enough that it can fit right in with your daily routine with little hassle. Sure, intermittent fasting does not produce results immediately, but you can keep fasting intermittently as long as you want. This leads to a steady weight loss that will help you immensely in the long run. You may not notice how much weight you have lost the first week or so. But six months or a year later, you would be surprised how much fat you have shredded and wonder why you did not try this out way earlier than you did.

Chapter 3: How Does Fasting Work?

The idea of purposely depriving yourself of food may sound ludicrous, but all diets consist of "eat less, move more". To put it brutally simple, every single diet regimen out there is all about calories in, calories out (CICO). However, there are many ways to achieve this. Some require you to eat extremely few calories in a few days, causing you to feel ill. When you get to eat again, you eat more than you should, triggering the yo-yo effect in which the body actually gains more weight than you have lost.

You see, if you deprive yourself of food for too long, your body goes into starvation mode. When that happens, your body's metabolism slows down significantly. You want to keep your metabolism rate high as it helps break down your body fat into energy, allowing you to lose weight and feel energetic. Unfortunately, when the body is deprived of food for too long, it goes into emergency mode to preserve the energy. This is actually very helpful in a survival situation, as you want to have as much energy as possible to survive without food. However, in terms of weight loss, this is not ideal. You will feel drained and when you eat the next time, you will take in more calorie than you would normally.

As mentioned earlier, intermittent fasting can be just as simple as skipping breakfast. It sounds brutally simple, and it is. By skipping an entire meal each day, you reduce the number of calories you consume weekly, even if you eat slightly larger meals for the rest of the day. Overall, you still consume fewer calories a day.

Your body also operates differently when you are eating compared to when you are not. When you eat a meal, your body usually spends a few hours breaking down that food and absorbing its nutrients. This creates readily-available energy which your body would use up rather than the fat that you have stored. This is especially true if you just ate something that is rich in sugar or carbohydrates because your body prefers to burn sugar for energy before any other source.

During the fasted state, which is the hours that your body is not consuming or digesting any food, it only has your body fat to burn for energy because it does not have any food to burn anymore. The same goes for working out in a fasted state. Your body is also forced to burn fat from your body as the only source of energy available because both glucose and glycogen are already depleted during the fasting phase and has not been replenished with a pre-workout meal. Since you want to burn fat, you need to remain in the fasted state for as long as possible without triggering the starvation mode. So, why does intermittent fasting work?

You see, our bodies react to energy consumption, as in eating food, by producing insulin. The more sensitive our body is to insulin, the more efficiently the body can consume food. The time when our body is most sensitive to insulin is after a period of fasting. This fluctuation in insulin production and sensitivity can help lead to weight loss and muscle creation. Moreover, your body will burn through glycogen (which is the starch stored in your muscles and liver that your body burns for energy when needed) when you train, which also leads to increased insulin sensitivity. Therefore, your body will break down and consume food much more efficiently if you have a meal after working out.

During that period, the food you eat will be converted to glycogen and stored in the muscles or burned as energy immediately to fuel the body and assist in the recovery process, leaving only a minuscule amount left to be stored as fat. When you compare this to a regular day without intermittent fasting, your insulin sensitivity will be at a normal level, and only a part of the energy generated from foods and carbs will be used immediately to fuel the body, with much more leftover to be stored as fat.

Moreover, growth hormone is also increased during the fastedstate, both during sleep and after a period phase. When you combine the increased growth hormone secretion and increased hormone sensitivity (by lowering insulin production), you are basically priming your body for muscle growth and fat loss with intermittent fasting.

Basically, intermittent fasting can help train your body to consume food much more efficiently by burning the fat it has already stored because you deprive it of new calories to derive energy from. Overall, there are many different physiological reasons why intermittent fasting helps promote weight loss and muscle growth if you do it properly.

Chapter 4: Why You Should Try IF

Intermittent fasting is natural for our body, as it is more used to periods of scarcity than abundance. As such, there are many health benefits associated with intermittent fasting such as:

Skin

Let's face it. Many of us have suffered from acne and regular breakouts throughout our teenage and adult years, even though you have been eating healthy and washing your face regularly. When you start pushing your first meal later into the day, your skin will improve gradually. Give your body enough time from digesting food and it will detox itself. Eating actually puts quite a lot of stress on the body, not the kind that triggers autophagy. The stress here will come out in many ways, one of which includes breaking out.

Improved Breathing

If you have short breaths at times, perhaps you should give IF a shot. We take breathing for granted until we no longer cannot breathe. When that happens, we soon realize how miserable life can be if you have short breaths. Of course, that is not to say that intermittent fasting alone helps improve your breathing condition. You may also need to cut out gluten, limiting dairy, and avoid secondhand smoking and fragrance.

Cravings

Craving for healthy food is not bad because it encourages you to eat healthily. It all boils down to how you control your cravings. If you crave pizzas and burgers, that's bad. If you crave salads, that's a good thing. You may experience this craving for healthy food when you start skipping breakfast. If you eat too many times a day regularly, you may take regular, healthy food for granted and start to crave junk food.

Cooking Skills

Later on we will discuss how you can combine intermittent fasting with other diets. Because the meals you may eat are often unavailable in many restaurants, you need to do your own cooking at home. Initially, this will be your biggest challenge if you have never cooked for yourself. However, consider this a learning opportunity as you may develop a strong appreciation for homemade meals.

Large Meals

Another great thing about intermittent fasting is that you can eat larger meals during the eating window. Every diet regimen all boils down to calorie in and calorie out. Because you create a calorie deficit by skipping breakfast, you can now eat more than you usually do. Of course, we recommend that you eat large healthy meals which calories do not exceed the deficit. This will leave you feeling more full and satisfied.

Weight Loss

This is the main reason why many people fast intermittently. Intermittent fasting acts as a powerful appetite suppressant, allowing you to control your eating habits more easily. As such, IF makes for a sound strategy for cutting fat. You will feel uneasy at first, but once your body adapts to the change, you will feel a sense of mental clarity and determination. Moreover, fasting lowers insulin, boosts HGH, and increases catecholamine. All of this puts you in the best fat-burning state. There will be no more stubborn body fat. You may even enjoy coffee more as the stimulant in coffee works more effectively.

Muscle Growth

Just by doing strength exercise three times a week, you may be able to pick up almost 10 pounds of muscle by fasting 16 hours every day. If you do most of your training on an empty stomach after ingesting about 10g of BCAA, which is to increase the protein synthesis and prevent protein breakdown, you can get this result as well. Of course, there are ways to maximize your muscle growth, and the basic idea is to bring in high carb and protein for your post-workout meal. When you fast, you increase your insulin sensitivity, which allows your body to break down food, store and use carbohydrates in your muscles.

Mental Clarity

Fasting also improves your mental clarity, allowing you to be more productive, determined, and have a better focus. Everything will seem clearer to you because your mind only needs to focus on what you are doing and not much else because digesting food is off the list.

Better Health

Well, of course, you would be healthier. Here, we mean that you would not catch common diseases as often, especially the common cold. Some people get sick very often, but they have reported that they do not become ill as often when they started fasting intermittently. Why? Because your body has the time to detoxify itself, allowing it to strengthen its immune system to protect you from diseases.

Libido

Okay, not a common subject to talk about, but men and women alike understand what it is to have a healthy libido. You can file this under mental clarity, but the reason why your libido is strengthened is that your hormone level is improved, especially for men because of their increased testosterone level.

Chapter 5: Fasting Regimens

Before we get to the fasting regimens you can incorporate into your daily life, let us take a quick detour to visit a bodily process known as autophagy. It is a pretty neat system in our body that can result from fasting.

Autophagy

You may be so sick of trying out juice cleanses and detox diets because you realize that they are nothing more than marketing bluffs to get you to buy their products using pseudoscience. Of course, you can drink your weight in liquid kale, but do not expect it to work any better than giving your body actual food. If anything, you are causing more damage to it than good. Instead of listening to the claims of juice cleanses and detox diets out there, you first need to know how your body cleans itself. Then, you can see through the lies of advertisements. The good news is that it is a process that you can control.

In short, autophagy is a process in which your cells create membranes that find, devour, and break up old, dead, or diseased cells. From that, whatever is usable is extracted and is used to create new, healthier cells. In simpler terms, it is your body recycling old, weak, and perhaps even cancerous cells, it uses whatever is left from the scrapped cell to create new, functional cells. Recycling is good, right?

According to Colin Champ, M.D., a board-certified radiation oncologist, assistant professor at the University of Pittsburgh Medical Center, and author of Misguided Medicine, autophagy allows your body to become more efficient with its resources immediately available by simply getting rid of faulty parts, prevent cancerous growth, and stop metabolic dysfunctions like diabetes and obesity.

There is also other evidence suggesting that autophagy also plays a role in controlling inflammation and immunity. This test was demonstrated on lab rats, and it is found that the ones that are incapable of autophagy tend to be lazier, slower, and are more susceptible to high cholesterol and even impaired brains. Therefore, we can conclude that autophagy is one way to slow down our aging process just by allowing our body to swap out old parts for new ones. You have three options to kick-start autophagy.

3 Ways to Autophagy

All three methods have one thing in common. Autophagy responds to stress, so all ofthe three methods will put stress on your body and force it into action.

Exercise

Unpleasant? Yes. Healthy? Indeed. Now you have another reason to keep exercising because all that sweating, grunting and post-workout pain will be worth it as exercise stresses your body. To develop muscle growth, you need to damage it by causing microscopic tears on your muscles. This causes your body to heal those wounds quickly, and consequently, make it stronger in order to prepare it for future damage you may expose them to. Many people do not realize that regular exercise is the most common way to cleanse the body, this is because it excretes toxins from the body through sweat. That is why you feel fresh after working out.

There is a study conducted on mice, they were engineered to have glowing green autophagosomes. These are the structures that form around cells that your body wants to recycle. When they glowed green, scientists were able to observe the cell recycling process of the body. They found that mice have a higher recycling rate after they ran for 30 minutes on a treadmill, compared to mice that are in a relaxed state. The rate was also even higher when the mice ran for 80 minutes. The result surprised the lead scientists so much so that they decided to purchase treadmills themselves.

However, you may argue that the study was conducted on mice, therefore, the results may not be applicable to humans. That is partially true, as of course we are very different to rodents. According to Daniel Klionsky, Ph.D., a cellular biologist at the University of Michigan, specializing in autophagy, it is hard to determine how much we need to exercise to get autophagy going. Still, there are many benefits of exercising other than autophagy, so regardless it is a good idea. If you love intense exercise to push your body to the limit, this is even better. Colin Champ recommends relatively intense exercises if you wish to maximize weight loss.

Fast

This is what this book is all about, and we have talked about it extensively. What we haven't told you is that fasting also stresses the body. If you have been on a juice cleanse, now is a good time to stop because it works against autophagy. You may not feel good when you fast, but at least it has many long-term health benefits.

In fact, fasting has been proven to have a lot of health benefits even when you only do it occasionally. Again, we have discussed this at great length in the previous chapters, and two of those benefits are lowered risks of diabetes and heart disease. Both of these might be related to autophagy.

Autophagy may also affect the brain, according to some research. This means that the risk of neurodegenerative diseases such as Parkinson's or Alzheimer's can be reduced. Other studies also showed that intermittent fasting improves cognitive function, brain structure, and neuroplasticity, meaning that it becomes easier to learn. Still, scientists have not been able to prove that autophagy is linked to all of this. Plus, the studies were only conducted on rodents. Therefore, we cannot assume that humans can gain all the same benefits.

Lower Your Carb Intake

There are plenty of ways to fast, and we will get to them very soon. Some people fast 18 hours a day a few times a week. That may be too much for beginners. A study published on 11 February 2011 on the multiple roles of autophagy in cancer showed that it is possible to achieve a lower risk of heart disease even if you only fast one day a month. Forgoing food occasionally seems to work, but there are other ways to get similar benefits without giving up eating comfort food.

Lowering your carb intake may result in ketosis, which is the current health and fitness trend alongside intermittent fasting. The idea here is to cut down on carbohydrates to a level low enough so the body has to burn the body's fat to fuel itself. So, ketosis is a good solution to weight loss without harming the muscles. There is some evidence suggesting that ketosis helps the body fight cancerous tumors, lower the risk of diabetes, and protects you against brain disorders, especially epilepsy. Additionally, another piece of research found that more than 50% of children suffering from epilepsyexperience at least a 50% reduction in seizures after going on the diet.

Ketosis can be considered to be an autophagy hack, according to Colin Champ. You can get the same metabolic changes and benefits from fasting without really fasting. However, keep in mind that keto diets are often high in fat. So, you need 60 to 70 percent of calorie intake to come from fat. That will mean a diet involving lots of steaks, bacon, and peanut butter shakes. Protein only makes up about 20 to 30 percent, and carbs are always below 50 grams a day.

However, if you find that staying in ketosis is harder than not eating altogether, there is an alternative. Similar benefits have been found in people following a diet with carbs not exceeding 30 percent of their overall calories.

Is There Any Other Way?

Unfortunately, these are the only three ways that are scientifically proven to trigger the autophagy process in your body. But here's the good news. Because intermittent fasting and autophagy are so sought after, there are incentives for scientists to work toward the use of pills to trigger autophagy. Currently, there may be some products out there that claim it can work wonders by triggering autophagy through its chemical substance. As with any online product people are trying to sell, it is worth checking the facts first. We understand that it is very tempting to buy pills that you can take to trigger autophagy so you do not have to purposely starve yourself. However, because research studies so far have only been conducted on rodents, we are still a long way from developing a reliable product, so we suggest you avoid it altogether.

There is even more good news here. We mentioned previously that ketosis was observed to have reduced epileptic seizures by half in children. There are also anti-epileptic drugs that are being developed that produce the same effects of ketosis. Should its development be successful and it is made available to the general public, it is possible that those pills are the key to trigger autophagy with no effort at all.

Whatever it is, try not to get your hopes up because there are just so many metabolic changes that occur during ketosis. Therefore, trying to match it with a pill may be near impossible. Perhaps it is necessary that we put our body through the stress that comes with ketosis in order to gain all the benefits.

However, while intermittent fasting means depriving yourself of sustenance, it does not have to be torture. You do not need to fast or remain in ketosis for too long or exercise intensely all day every day to reap all of those benefits. Just a few hours of any of the above is good enough to get autophagy going.

With autophagy out of the way, let us discuss how you can trigger this effect using various intermittent fasting methods.

The 16:8 Method

The most common fasting method of them all is the 16:8 IF. It is the most basic and practiced form of IF. Here, you need to fast for 16 hours and eat in the remaining 8-hour window. Sounds simple, right?

You need to stick to the hours, but there is no need to count the seconds. This method is good for beginners as it is very easy to do. There is also a variation that you can follow if this is too difficult, as it can be if you have not done fasting before. Ladies tend to struggle in this regard, so you can alter it for a bit. You can start by fasting for only 12 hours at a time, which is very easy considering that you sleep for 8 hours, so the remaining 4 should be a breeze. Then, you can step it up to 14-hour fast and eventually 16 when you are more familiar with it. Of course, since the 16:8 method is the easiest, it has its drawback for not being as effective compared to other methods. Still, the body has more than enough time to cleanse itself.

The main reason why this method is preferred, even among IF veterans, is the fact that you still receive enough food every day. You will not starve for a long time. You will spend about half of the fasting period sleeping if you sleep for 8 hours a day (and you should). Everyone could survive with one less meal a day.

Here's a tip: eating the right food helps. We mentioned that you can eat normally in intermittent fasting. That is true, but you can optimize your weight-loss even further. You should eat high-fat food or eggs as the last meal before fasting. If you eat something sweet, then the food is quickly turned into glucose. In your body, this means that the blood sugar level rises rapidly. As a result, your body releases insulin and the blood sugar level drops again, but it will also drop below its normal value, and then you quickly have another craving for sweets.

In the end, if you eat something greasy or eggs, then your stomach and your intestines will take longer to digest. This gives you longer feeling full. Then, you are less hungry and can easily survive fasting.

How you arrange the hours of fasting and eating is entirely up to you, only 16 (or 14) hours must be in one go. There are several possible combinations. Let's say you skip breakfast. Then your first meal of the day is your lunch, and you have it at 12. Then you have something smaller such as a coffee, then you have dinner at 8. Then, eat eggs or something fried, and go to bed a few hours later. In the morning, you get up, skip breakfast, drink some coffee, water or tea, and then go to work. But we advise against drinking coffee because if you drink too much, your body will become overstimulated and will leave you feeling hungry.

If you follow this routine, you will feel better in the morning, a lot more energetic. Eventually, you will no longer feel the cravings for food. Before you know it, it is already noon and you can enjoy lunch. Congratulations, you just fasted for 16 hours successfully.

As we have mentioned earlier, fasting and eating can be flexible. So, if you prefer to eat in the morning, you can still be flexible with your time. So, you can start fasting at 3 in the afternoon and then stop at 7 am the next day, and start the day with breakfast. After breakfast, you have lunch at 12 pm. Because the time of fasting and eating are not set in stone, you can time your fasting and eating phase as you want, just make sure that they are done in one go, as in fasting for 16 hours straight, not 8 hours, then eat, and then fast for another 8 hours. Consider trying out different times so you know what works best. Then, stick to it so your body can get used to it, therefore you will not feel as hungry.

When you fast, it is important to keep yourself hydrated. Avoid alcohol, sweet drinks, etc. Unsweetened tea, water, and coffee (no milk or sugar) are fine. Make sure to drink these regularly and you will feel better.

Sometimes, it can be tricky to get into the rhythm from the start, especially if you are new to the whole IF methods. Here, it is possible to get used to fasting slowly by first deciding when you want to fast and when you want to eat. Suppose that you want to fast from 8 pm to 12 pm. Then, you start having breakfast a little later in increments. If you usually eat at 7 am, then you move it to 7:30 am. At the same time, you are putting lunch a little bit back. So you bring the two meals closer together until they overlap. Then move that eating time slowly to lunch time and voila, you are now in your 16:8 rhythm.

The Crescendo Method

The Crescendo method is well-known for its effectiveness for women who want to try out intermittent fasting. As mentioned previously, the female body responds to IF differently from men, and the side effects can be nasty. Therefore, alternative methods are created. The Crescendo Method is one of them, being an alteration of the 16:8 method by fasting for only 12 hours as opposed to 16. This method is a gentle way to get women into intermittent fasting, which is perfect for ladies as it does not rub their hormones in the wrong way.

The main reason why it is great for ladies and beginners alike is the fact that it is realistic. You do not need to fast for 16 hours a day. 12 hours is good enough. You can have dinner at 8 PM and breakfast at 8 AM, it's like a normal day. You fast for 12 hours. It is easy to get into this routine.

There is no need to fast daily. You can be flexible with the days you want to spend fasting. You just need to spend a few non-consecutive days fasting every week, and you are good to go! So, you can eat normally on a Monday because Monday is horrible and you want to make it as least horrible as possible. Then, you do that again on Wednesday. Then, you eat normally on a Friday because you might want to enjoy your Friday night and the weekend. You fast for 12 hours on Tuesday, Thursday, Saturday, and Sunday. Voila! You have a perfect week.

Even though this method of fasting is gentle, it is still shown that it can reduce body fat, lessen inflammation, and improve your energy.

There are some tips we would like to give you to help you get into the routine. First, you should alternate the days you fast. Try not to have consecutive eating days like Monday to Wednesday and then fast for the rest of the week. You might feel horrible at the end of the week. Some people fast on Tuesday, Thursday, and Saturday, but we found that fasting on Monday, Wednesday, and Friday works the best for many people as you can have the whole weekend to rest. Still, it's worth experimenting and sticking to what works best for you. Again, try not to have consecutive fasting days.

On those fasting days, try to do some low-intensity workout, if you do exercise (and you probably should). We will discuss how exercise can be useful for intermittent fasting in a later chapter. It is also worth mentioning that you should eat healthy food every day, get in enough water, about 64 ounces, every day.

Now, if you are starting out and are unsure about this whole fasting method, you can start small. Start with one day of fasting a week, then bump it up to two and then three when you are ready.

The One Meal a Day Method(OMAD)

The OMAD method is also a commonly used method and is considered to be one of the hardest methods out there. Basically, you fast only once or twice a week but 24 hours at a time. Then, on the other days, you can eat normally. Whatever eating pattern you eat is entirely up to you, just make sure you eat responsibly.

Still, it is a bad idea to not eat the entire day. You should schedule your time in a way that you can have a meal every day, and still fast in-between. That means you should not fast from Monday morning before breakfast to Tuesday. Instead, have dinner at 8 on a Monday and fast until dinnertime at 8 on a Tuesday. That way, you still eat something every day and fast at the same time. You need that energy to get through the day, after all.

The OMADmethod is different from the previous two methods because you need to fast for longer periods of time,therefore, it is worth looking into how it works. When you reduce the eating window, you create a larger fasting period. During this time, the body will use up the stored glycogen created from carbohydrates. When that is burned up, the body goes into a ketogenic state and burns fat for fuel. This basically translates to you losing weight. As you can probably guess, the OMAD method is simply a twist to the existing IF methods.

The good thing about the OMAD method is the fact that you only restrict your calorie intake once or twice a week or every other day. You can eat normally for the rest of the week. Since you fast for 24 hours, we recommend you break your fast with light, easily digestible and nutritious foods. Plus, you can be flexible with your time, meaning that you can start fasting at 6 in the morning or 10 in the evening – whatever works best for you. Of course, you should time it so that you have at least one meal a day.

Because you need to fast only once or twice a week, you can fit it into your life very easily along with other routines such as; working out, parties, working, family, etc., compared to other methods where a family gathering means you're having a cheat day. Moreover, you do not necessarily have to starve yourself for 24 hours. You can help yourself with some green tea or black coffee, and have some solid food such as an egg or an apple during the day. That way, you will not blackout from the lack of food. You don't want that to happen when you are driving. Therefore, it is wise to ensure your own safety first since everybody is unique and responds differently to even the same fasting method. The OMAD method is probably for you if you want to try something different. It is arguably easier for beginners as well because they just need to focus on fasting once or twice a week. It helps if you fast on the days when you are busiest because all the work you need to do will help shift your focus away from the hunger. Otherwise, you can fast on a weekend day because you do not need as much energy if you stay in. You can rest to compensate for the lack of food, and you can distract yourself from the hunger with things you like to do.

The OMAD method also has its own downsides. Of course, not eating 24 hours at a time can be tough for some people and it can actually increase the likelihood of binging when the fasting is over, which defeats the purpose of fasting. There is no point in restricting your calorie intake once or twice a week if you are just going to overeat for the rest of the week to compensate for the calories lost.

The OMAD method works only if you are willing to go the long stretch of fasting at a time, and can control yourself from not overeating for the rest of the week. It might not be for you if you often need to go out with your friends and family. Another thing that we should point out is that, if you have any medical complications, we advise you to talk to your doctor before you start any new eating plan, including intermittent fasting.

While OMAD requires you to restrict your calorie intake for almost 24 hours at a time, it is worth pointing out that it will not work if you do not control what you eat. You may be surprised to know that all that 24 hours of progress will be for nothing if you eat uncontrollably for that one-hour window. So, what do you need when you are on the OMAD diet?

OMAD and Exercise

At first, when you fast for an extended period of time, your body will need to adjust and you may feel exhausted, meaning you are unable to exercise. This is normal. Even if you attempt to exercise, the fatigue may weaken you so much that you cannot put enough effort into doing it properly, which could result in serious injuries in some cases. Your body has not been fed for a long time, and so your muscles are also weakened. To keep your muscles active, start light by doing stretching exercises or yoga first.

From there, as your body starts to adjust to the new eating routine, you can slowly introduce muscle toning workouts to prevent the sagging of your skin. Of course, you should always consult a qualified and competent trainer to design a workout that suits you, while accounting for your medical condition and body type. Whether you go on theOMADdiet or not, you should always practice meditation everyday through the traditional method, or when you are out walking or running.

Risks and Cautions

There are a few things you need to know if you are just starting out. Even when you have been using the 16:8 method, extending your fasting period to almost 24 hours and leaving yourself with little room to eat can still be tricky.

When you first start this diet plan, you will feel hungry and restless. Do not panic. This is natural. You may feel dizzy and experience brain fog along the way too, especially towards the end of your fasting phase. You might not be able to concentrate properly and metabolism in menopausal women may slow down.

Because our bodies respond differently to the same diets, it is absolutely necessary that you consult your doctor or a registered dietitian before you start following this diet. Moreover, pregnant or lactating women should not try this diet.

Alternate-Day Fasting

Alternate-Day fasting is another alteration to the existingOMADmethod. Here, the idea is that you fast for 24 hours, eat the next 24 hours, and fast again the next day. During fasting days, you can drink as many calorie-free drinks as you want such as; water, unsweetened tea, and coffee.

If this is too difficult for you, you can alter it even further by eating only 500 calories a day on fasting days, or roughly 20% to 25% of your energy requirements. This again creates a calorie deficit but not so much that you would feel dizzy. You can still achieve the weight loss benefits regardless of whether you consume calories at lunch, dinner, or as small meals throughout the day, as they don't seem to make any difference. As always, everyone varies, so you may find that one of the previous methods works better for you than ADF. Because you get to consume something during the fasting day to keep your body going, the modified version of ADF is a lot more sustainable than doing full fasts on fasting days and it is just as effective anyway.

Health Benefits

ADF has been proven to have many other health benefits such as:

Type 2 Diabetes

95% of diabetes cases are type 2 diabetes. Moreover, one in three Americans are obese and have pre-diabetes. Pre-diabetes, as the name suggests, is a condition in which the blood sugar rises higher than normal but not so high that it can be considered diabetic. Even so, pre-diabetes is just one step away from diabetes. Therefore, you need to take control of your blood sugar level. A great way to improve your health andreverse many debilitating symptoms of type 2 diabetes is by losing weight and restricting calories.

Similarly to continuous calorie restriction, ADF weakens the risk factors associated with type 2 diabetes among overweight and obese individuals. This fasting method works the best in lowering insulin levels and reducing insulin resistance without disrupting the blood sugar control system, which is super effective because high insulin levels are linked to obesity and many other chronic diseases such as cancer and heart disease. A fasting regimen lasting between 8 to 12 weeks under the ADF method has shown to decrease insulin by 30% among pre-diabetic individuals.

In short, the reduction in insulin levels and insulin resistance may reduce the risk of type 2 diabetes altogether, especially when you lose weight at the same time.

Heart Health

Heart disease is the bane of mankind, being one of the leading causes of death in the world at 25% or 1 in four deaths. When you think about it, dying to a heart attack is one of the worst ways to go because it may strike out of the blue, and there is only so much you can do to prepare for the sudden strike. A lot of studies show that ADF is a good solution for overweight and obese people to lose weight while also reducing heart disease risk factors. Again, a test lasted between 8 to 12 weeks under the ADF methods with obese and overweight individuals as subjects. The study found that ADF may yield common health benefits such as:

- Smaller waist circumference (5-7 cm or 2-3 in of reduction)
- Decreased blood pressure
- Decreased blood triglycerides (Up to 30%)
- Lowered cholesterol concentration (20-25%)
- Increased number of large LDL-particles and reduction in dangerous small, dense LDL particles

Autophagy and ADF

ADF also has a special interaction with autophagy, which we will get to in a later chapter. ADF stimulates autophagy, which is a process in which old parts of your cells are recycled and replaced with better ones. So, your body can prevent diseases such as cancer, neurodegeneration, heart disease, and other infections. Studies on animals have shown that both long-term and short-term fasting increase autophagy. Plus, are linked to a delay in aging and reduced risk of tumors.

Moreover, fasting has also been shown to increase lifespan in rodents, flies, yeasts, and worms. As far as we know, human studies have shown that ADF does reduce oxidative damage and promote changes that may be linked to longevity. Of course, you should not expect that you will live longer by a significant margin, but you can take comfort in knowing that at least you will live healthier with ADF.

Starvation Mode and ADF

Most weight reduction strategies cause a slight drop in resting metabolic rate, and high metabolic rate is the thing that we need to keep up here. This drop is known as the starvation mode, yet the specialized term is versatile thermogenesis.

When you limit your calories, your body will endeavor to save vitality by decreasing the number of calories it consumes. Your body does not really need to consume a similar measure of calories consistently to work. Consider it the battery sparing mode. You may feel somewhat languid, however, you don't tire as fast. In any case, that is the issue. At the point when your body does not consume the same number of calories, you quit getting in shape while likewise making you feel hopeless. Here, ADF does not appear to cause a drop in metabolic rate.

There was an investigation that contrasted ADF with standard calorie confinement more than about two months, and the outcomes demonstrated that constant calorie limitation causes a significant drop in resting metabolic rate by 6%, while ADF just purposes a little plunge of 1%. Additionally, following 24 unsupervised weeks, the subjects that experienced standard calorie limitation still had a 4.5% lower resting metabolic rate contrasted with before the examination, though the ADF subjects kept up their unique metabolic rate. Numerous impacts related to ADF might be in charge of keeping up a moderately high metabolic rate, including the preservation of bulk.

Is It a Good Idea?

ADF has its uses outside weight-loss. It also has many health benefits even for normal-weight people. A 3-week study conducted on individuals with normal-weight who follow a strict ADF diet, with zero calories on fasting days, showed increased fat burning rate, decreased fasting insulin rate, and a 4% decrease in fat mass. However, subjects reported that they felt hungry throughout the study. That is why you should consider following the ADF diet with one small meal on fasting days, as it is more tolerable for normal-weight people.

Another controlled study on both normal-weight and overweight individuals showed that, after following ADF diet for 12 weeks, it resulted in reduced fat mass and favorable changes in risk factors associated with heart disease. Here, it is worth pointing out that the reason why you lose weight is the fact that ADF normally gives you much fewer calories than you need to maintain weight. If you do not want to lose weight or fat mass in the first place, then ADF may not be for you, and other dietary methods will most likely suit you better.

Drinks

There is no general rule when it comes to what you should eat or drink on fasting days, except that it should not exceed 500 calories in total. So, it is best to drink low or calorie-free drinks on fasting days, such as water, coffee, and tea. Many people find it best to eat a large meal late in the day, while others prefer eating early or split the meal between 2 to 3 meals, all within 500 calories.

Because your calorie intake will be limited, you should make sure you get the 500 calories from nutritious, high-protein foods, as well as low-calorie vegetables. That way, you will feel full without consuming too many calories. You should also consider trying out soups because they tend to make you feel fuller than if you eat the ingredients separately.

Here are a few ideas of what you should eat during fasting days:

- Lots of salad with lean meat
- Soup and piece of fruit
- Grilled fish or lean meat with vegetables
- Yogurt with berries
- Eggs and vegetables

There are also plenty of quick 500-calorie meals and healthy low-calorie snacks out there. All you need to do is a quick Google search. As always, make sure to check if you have any allergies to any of the ingredients. You do not want to have a nasty surprise while you are fasting.

Is It Safe?

The final verdict. According to numerous studies, ADF is shown to be safe for most people. Quite contrary to belief, ADF does not result in a greater risk of weight regain compared to traditional, calorie-restricted diets. On the other hand, ADF may be better for long-term weight loss compared to continuous calorie restriction.

Some believe that ADF heightens risks of overeating or binge eating, but studies have shown that it actually decreased depression and binge eating. It also improved restrictive eating and body image perception among obese individuals.

Of course, we said that ADF is shown to be safe with most people because there are always groups of people who should not adhere to any weight loss diet. So, consult your doctor before you start changing up your diet plans, especially if you have a medical condition or are currently taking any medications. These groups include people with eating disorders, pregnant and lactating mothers, children and underweight individuals or those who have certain medical conditions.

The 5:2 Diet

The 5:2 diet, which is also known as the Fast Diet, is one of the easiest fasting diets. This diet got its name because you will get five days a week eating normally and the other two are restricted to 500-600 calories a day. Similar to a few other intermittent fasting methods, what matters here is when you eat your meals, not what you eat. So, this is more of a lifestyle than a diet regimen. A lot of people find that this is easier than a traditional calorie-restricted diet.

It is very simple to follow. You fast for 2 nonconsecutive days and consume 500 calories if you are a woman, and 600 calories if you are a man. What days you fast do not matter, just make sure that there is at least one non-fasting day in between them.

If losing weight is your priority, then the 5:2 diet can prove to be very effective if done properly. This is because the 5:2 method helps you consume fewer calories without putting too much stress on your body. The weight loss comes when you fast for those two days, and the lack of calories will force your body to consume the fat in your body while still providing enough so that your body does not eat up your muscles or slow down your metabolism to preserve energy. Because you will only lose weight during the two fasting days, it is critical that you do not compensate for the calories you missed during the fasting days by eating more on non-fasting days.

This method will not work if you compensate for the calories you missed. That said, fasting methods similar to the 5:2 diet have shown a lot of promise in weight loss studies:

- A recent review discovered that modified alternate-day fasting led to weight loss of 3 to 8% over 3 to 24 weeks.
- In the same study, participants have reported that their waist circumference has shrunk by 4 to 7%, meaning that they have lost a lot of harmful belly fat.
- Intermittent fasting causes a significant reduction in muscle mass compared to other weight loss with conventional calorie restriction.
- Combined with exercises, intermittent fasting is even more effective, such as endurance or strength training. We will discuss this in more details later.

Eating During Fasts

There is no rule for what or when you should eat on fasting days here, unlike the 16:8 method. Some people find it more convenient to start their day with a small breakfast. Others find that eating as late as possible is better. Normally though, there are two meal patterns that people follow.

You can have three meals a day as usual, but the amount of calories is divided between those three meals. So, if you are a man, you can divide your 600 calories over three meals. You'd have 200 calories for breakfast, lunch, and dinner equally. That, or you could have a 300-calorie breakfast, 200-calorie lunch, and 100-calorie dinner. Again, it is up to you to decide how you want to portion your limited number of calories throughout the day, although it may be a good idea to start off strong with a relatively large breakfast, smaller lunch, and smallest dinner as you may not need to spend as much energy at the end of the day. The same applies if you are a woman, although you will only have 500 calories to work with so divide them wisely. You can have somewhat balanced meals of 250-calorie breakfast, 150-calorie lunch, and 150-calorie dinner. That or prioritize getting most out of your breakfast with 300-calorie breakfast, and 100-calorie lunch and dinner. Again, experiment and find out what works best for you and stick to it.

Another approach is to have two slightly larger meals instead of three. The same principle applies, except that you only get to eat twice. Whatever you do, remember that your calorie intake is limited – 600 for men and 500 for women. So, it is best to use your calorie budget wisely. It is best to make the most out of your calorie intake, so we suggest that you go for nutritious, high-fiber, high-protein foods that make you feel full without consuming too many calories. As mentioned previously, soups are a great option. A few examples of healthy foods such as, still or sparkling water, tea, black coffee, low-calorie cup soups, soups (miso, tomato, cauliflower or vegetables), lots of vegetables, boiled or baked eggs, grilled fish or lean meat, natural yogurt with berries, or cauliflower rice.

Again, there is no one-size-fits-all meals here, so you need to experiment a bit to find out what works for you and stick to it.

What if I feel Ill?

If you are new to fasting and intermittent fasting, expect to experience moments of great hunger. This is to be expected. You might also feel weak or slow. However, hunger will eventually fade, especially if you try to distract yourself with work or other things. Fasters have reported that the fasting gets easier the more they do it. You certainly are going to be alright eventually.

However, there is no need to turn this into torture. Intermittent fasting is highly customizable. So, if you are not used to fasting, it may be best to keep some small snacks handy during your first few fasts, just in case you feel unwell.

Still, if the problem persists and you continue to feel ill or faint during fast days, eat something and consult with your doctor about whether you should continue. While fasting is highly personal, there are some people who cannot do it because of medical conditions. Fasting is very safe or healthy for many people, but everyone varies. It does not suit everyone. It is more intended for healthy, well-nourished individuals. Some people should avoid fasting or any other dietary restrictions completely, including:

- Pregnant women, nursing mothers, teenagers, children and people with type 1 diabetes
- Individuals who often experience drops in sugar levels
- Individuals with a history of eating disorders
- Individuals who are malnourished, underweight, or have known nutrient deficiencies
- Women who have fertility issues or are trying to conceive

Which One Should I Follow?

Looking at all of the options above, you are spoiled for choice. The rule of thumb is to try them all and see which regimen works for you. Most people have a busy schedule so they pick one that fits into the schedule perfectly so there is no need to move things around to accommodate the lifestyle change. If you have plenty of time on your hand, we suggest you work your way up starting from the Crescendo method, then 16:8, then 5:2, then OMAD, then ADF. We have arranged them in order of supposed difficulty.

Chapter 6: What Shall I Eat?

Similar to exercising, intermittent fasting only works if you eat the right kind of food. You need to make sure that you eat healthy food that gives you enough calories and makes you feel full. Here, we will discuss some of the foods you should consider including in your diet alongside your fasting regimen so you can optimize your weight loss without compromising your health.

Good Food

You should eat kale, spinach, white peek potato, sweet potato, bell peppers, lettuce, Chinese cabbage, violet cabbage, scallions, turnip, beetroot, cauliflower, cabbage, broccoli and carrot for veggies.

For fruits, acai berries, gooseberries, blueberries, strawberries, pineapple, tangerine, lime, lemon, plum, peach, tomato, cucumber, grapefruit, orange, banana, apple, and a limited number of mangoes should be eaten.

For your protein fix, your options include eggs, tofu, beans and legumes, mushroom, fish, lean cuts of pork and beef, and chicken breast.

As for your diary, you can choose from cottage cheese, homemade ricotta cheese, buttermilk, feta cheese, cheddar cheese, full-fat yogurt, and full-fat milk.

As for fats and oils, you have almond butter, peanut butter, sunflower butter, olive oil, rice bran oil, and edible grade coconut oil.

If you love eating nuts and seeds, you can eat melon seeds, pumpkin seeds, sunflower seeds, macadamia, pistachios, pine nuts, pecan, almond, and walnut.

As for herbs and spices, you have clove, garlic powder, cardamom, star anise, allspice, chili flakes, white pepper, black pepper, cayenne pepper, turmeric, cumin, coriander, onion, ginger, garlic, oregano, thyme, rosemary, fennel, dill, mint, and cilantro.

Finally, for something to wet your mouth, you can go for water, homemade lemonade or electrolyte, coconut water, cold-pressedjuices,and freshly pressed fruit juice.

As you can probably tell, you are already spoiled for choice here, even when you fast. With these, you can cook up some delectable dishes for yourself as a reward for your hard work. Of course, these are generally what you should eat. We also want to point out some of the things you need to avoid to maintain your health.

Overall, I advocate just eating a healthy and balanced diet,it can be adjusted to meet your goals. Of course, don't limit yourself to this list, generally, we know what is good for our body and what isn't. However, certain things will differ for everyone.

For example, someone trying to gain muscle will have different nutritional needs to someone who is trying to lose weight, therefore, in terms of macronutrients and calories I highly recommend deciding what your goals are and using calculators as well as your own research to discover what you need to eat in order to reach those goals.

It is also a similar story depending on your dietary preferences. A vegan will have a very different diet in order to meet all their nutritional needs to someone who eats animal products. Again, this requires more research depending on your goals, dietary preferences, current health,etc. There are many factors that go into this so it would be reductionist to say there is a one size fits all way to eat.

Bad Food

When it comes to fruit, you need to avoid fruits rich in GI such as grapes, jackfruit, pineapples, and mangoes. You can eat them but limit your intake.

As for protein, avoid fatty cuts of beef and pork, and bacon (especially bacon).

For dairy products, avoid low-fat milk, low-fat yogurt, cream cheese, and flavored yogurt.

You should also avoid whole grains such as white rice. Consume it in limited quantity and always eat it with at least five other veggies in the previous list to balance it out with the GI.

For fat and oils, avoid mayonnaise, margarine, butter, vegetable oil, lard, dalda, and hemp seed oil.

Also, avoid processed foods such as salami, ranch dip, sausages, fries, jellies, and bottled jams. Of course, It goes without saying processed takeaways are of course part of this list.

As for beverages, avoid packaged fruit and vegetable juices, soda, diet soda (it doesn't help), and energy drinks.

This is not to say that you absolutely have to cut out all the food above. Of course, you can enjoy treats every now and then, but as a general rule try and aim for 80% of the food you eat contribute to making you healthier and feel great. Certain types of fasting certainly give you leeway when it comes to food choices, but in terms of longevity and micronutrient intake, it is definitely best to develop a healthy and balanced diet.

Now that you know what to avoid, let us discuss how you could design your meal so that you do not lose your head while dieting.

What to Include in Your Meals

Consider this a general guide as to what a meal should look like to you.

- Five types of veggies
- Three types of fruits
- Lean protein, but you can eat some red meat once in a while
- Lots of plant protein like kidney beans, seeds, nuts, garbanzo beans, and whole pulses (if you are a vegetarian)
- A few unsalted nuts, only a few
- A piece of 80% dark chocolate, if you need to
- Fruits, sour cream, or yogurt if you want some more sweet treats
- Alternatively, you can bake and store brownies that have healthy ingredients and less sugar
- Keep yourself hydrated – you limit your calorie intake, not your fluid intake; stay well hydrated as this is one of the only things that keeps you going
- Alternatively, you can drink three or four cups of green tea during your fasting period

These are just some simple guidelines, but as we previously mentioned the overall goal is developing a healthy lifestyle that is sustainable to you, allows you to meet all your nutritional needs and achieve all your personal goals, whether that be weight loss or athletic performance. Therefore, further research is recommended depending on your situation. For example, if you are a vegan we would highly recommend checking out a complete vegan nutrition guide to make sure you know how to optimize your diet, the same goes for a meat eater as well, as in the modern world there are so many foods that are detrimental to our health an analysis of what we consume on a daily basis is definitely required.

This may sound like a lot of work, however, understanding what you put in your body and why is essential to developing a long term sustainable lifestyle, which is key to long term weight loss and health and is,therefore, certainly worth the time and effort required. As many have said across the ages, our health is our greatest wealth.

We will talk more about exercise in a later chapter, but you may already be wondering if you should consider working out when you are dieting, especially during an intense diet such as the OMAD method. After all, you do not eat for almost 24 hours, so surely you would feel tired at the end of the day – both mentally and physically. Exercising would only push yourself further, you may argue. The short answer is that you should. There will be more details in a later chapter.

Other Food Ideas

In addition to all of the previous food we have mentioned, here are some more food ideas you should consider including in your diet.

Filling Food

Different kinds of food make you feel full differently. For instance, a tub of rice is infinitely more filling than a tub of ice-cream. However, the calorie intake is also different. Rice has lower calories than ice-cream for the same food weight. We would eat less food if we feel full faster. So, try eating filling food to ward off hunger, allowing you to eat fewer calories at the next meal. But what makes a food filling?

The satiety index was created in 1995 to grade how filling a particular food is. To measure this, a study of 240-calorie servings of 38 different foods were tested. On this scale, foods were ranked based on their ability to sate hunger. Food with a score higher than 100 means it is more filling. That means you can cut down on your calorie intake by eating food that scores higher than 100. Of course, no one has the time to break out their calculator and satiety index chart. You can determine how filling the food is based on the following characteristics:

- Low in energy density: Food that is low in energy density has few calories for its weight. They are often very filling and they normally contain a lot of water and fiber, which is great for intermittent fasting as you need the water from food as well. Moreover, these kinds of foods are also low in fat.

- High in volume: Similarly, look for food that contains a lot of water or air as this may score high on the satiety index as well.

- High in fiber: Fiber gives substance, which is the bulk in the food that you eat, allowing you to feel full for longer by slowing down the emptying of the stomach and increase digestion time.

- High in protein: According to some studies, protein is the most filling macronutrient and that it changes the levels of many satiety hormones like ghrelin and GLP-1, allowing you to feel full faster and longer.

- As a rule of thumb, whole, unprocessed foods are usually more filling than processed foods.

As such, filling food should be incorporated into your diet plan so you can lose more weight in the long run. Here, we will look at 15 filling foods you should try out.

Boiled Potatoes

Potatoes, though bland, are very nutritious and is a staple food other than rice. Cooked, unpeeled potatoes have many minerals and vitamins such as potassium and vitamin C. Since potatoes are rich in water and carbs while containing a moderate amount of fiber and protein, as well as almost no fat, potatoes are very filling compared to many other high-carb foods. In fact, boiled potatoes snatch the first place on the satiety index at the score of 323, which is 7 times higher than croissants, which is the lowest on the satiety index.

A study found that eating boiled potatoes with pork steak result in lower calorie intake for the meal compared to combining it with white rice or pasta. A protein proteinase inhibitor 2 (PI2) which may suppress appetite is also found in potatoes, according to some evidence, making them more filling (NCBI: 2255726, 20820171).

Eggs

Eggs are also healthy as they are full of nutrients. Most of them are found in the yolks, which is where the chick draws its nutrients from as it develops and hatches. Antioxidants lutein and zeaxanthin that are beneficial to the eyes are also present in the yolk as well. Overall, eggs are a great source of protein as a large egg alone has up to six grams of protein, including all the nine essential amino acids. Plus, eggs also score fairly high on the satiety index, meaning that they are filling as well.

A study (NCBI: 16373948) found that eating eggs for breakfast instead of a bagel may increase your fullness and result in fewer calorie intake over the next 36 hours. Another study (NCBI: 23446906) also found that breakfast rich in protein, which includes eggs and lean beef, increases fullness and helps people make better food choices.

Oatmeal

Oatmeal is also a popular choice for breakfast. Because it is low in calories and high in fiber, especially beta-glucan, that is a soluble fiber, not to mention that it can soak up water, oats are ranked third place on the satiety index.

According to a study (NCBI: 26273900), participants reported feeling full and less hungry after eating oatmeal, compared to breakfast cereal. Subjects also ate fewer calories during lunch. Soluble fiber like the beta-glucan in oats, may make you feel full quicker and also cause your body to release satiety hormones and delay the emptying of the stomach (NCBI: 19753601, 19917449, 21115081).

Fish

Fish is also a great source of high-quality protein and is rich in omega-3 fatty acids, which are essential fats that we need from food. According to a study, omega-3 fatty acids may increase the feeling of fullness in overweight or obese people (NCBI: 18602429). Moreover, other studies suggest that the protein found in fish may have a stronger effect on fullness compared to any other sources of protein (NCBI: 7498104).

On the satiety index, fish scored the highest compared to any other protein-rich foods, including eggs and beef. Fish is ranked third out of the 38 foods tested. Another study also compared the protein found in fish, chicken, and beef. Researchers found that the protein found in fish has the most powerful effect on satiety (NCBI: 1542005).

Soups

While the evidence is mixed (NCBI: 14649371, 15639159), common sense dictates that liquids are often less filling than solid food. Soups, however, are a different story. Research (NCBI: 23818981, 23093339) shows that soups might be more filling than solid meals containing the same ingredients. In a study (NCBI: 23093339), volunteers consume a solid meal, a chunky soup, or a smooth soup that went through a food processor. From there, the feeling of fullness is measured as well as the rate of which the food left the stomach. Smooth soup had the biggest impact on fullness and is the slowest to leave the stomach, followed by the chunky soup.

Meat

Lean meats are also very filling. Beef scores 176 on the satiety index and it has a very powerful effect on satiety. In terms of protein content, beef is ranked right after fish. According to a study published in 1990 on NCBI (2228407) found that people who consume high-protein meat at lunch ate 12% less at dinner compared to those who had a high-carb lunch.

Greek Yogurt

Greek yogurt is very thick and rich in protein compared to regular yogurt. It is a great alternative to eggs as a breakfast option. Plus, it is also a popular afternoon snack that may make you feel full up until dinner, which allows you to eat less. According to a study published in 2013 on NCBI (23022602) conducted on women, subjects consumed a 160-

calorie yogurt that was low, moderate, or high in protein. Subjects who consumed high-protein Greek yogurt reported feeling full the longest and ate dinner at a later time compared to those who consumed lower calorie yogurt.

Vegetables

Vegetables are also nutritious because they contain all sorts of vitamins, minerals, and many other plant compounds that are beneficial to your health. Since they are rich in water content and low in calories, not to mention full of fiber, you will feel full eating these. Of course, the only downside is that vegetables are not as delicious, but they still are very satisfying to chew. A study published in 2004 on NCBI (15389416) shows that a large salad before a meal of pasta increases the feeling of fullness and reduces the calorie intake for that meal.

Cottage Cheese

Cottage cheese is also low in fat and carbs and dense in protein. Because high-protein food helps you feel full quicker even when you only consume a few calories, cottage cheese is also a great option. It is also just as filling as eggs.

Legumes

Legumes such as peas, lentils, peanuts, and beans are also very nutritious. They are loaded with fiber and plant-based protein and low in energy density. An article (NCBI: 24820437) reviewed nine randomized trails that observe post-meal fullness using pulses which are a part of the legume family, they found that subjects feel 31% more full in comparison to eating pasta and bread.

Fruit

Just like vegetables, fruits also have a low energy density. Rich in fiber, eating fruits will make you feel full as your body digests them slower. On the satiety index, apples and oranges score around 200. Here, it is worth pointing out that eating fruits and drinking fruit juices are two different things. The latter is very unhealthy, not to mention not very filling.

Quinoa

Quinoa is also another great source of protein. In fact, it contains all the essential amino acids your body needs. So, it is a viable source of protein. It also scores higher than most grains, so it is also a good option to keep you feel full and consume fewer calories.

Nuts

While we are talking about grains, nuts such as walnuts and almonds are also dense in energy and nutrients. Their size makes them a perfect snack option as an alternative to chips. As they are full of healthy fats and proteins, they are filling as well. In fact, a study (NCBI: 19144727) shows that chewing almonds only 40 times will greatly reduce your hunger and increase your feeling of fullness, compared to chewing for 10 or 25 times. So, have some almonds handy and start counting.

Coconut Oil

Coconut oil contains a special combination of fatty acids that are about 90% saturated. It consists mostly of medium-chain triglycerides and these fatty acids turn into ketone bodies when they enter the liver from the digestive tract. According to some studies (NCBI: 17228046), ketone bodies can reduce your appetite. Another study reported that individuals who eat breakfast with medium-chain triglycerides consume much fewer calories at lunch (NCBI: 9701177). Another study also looks at the effect of long-chain triglycerides and medium-chain triglycerides. According to the researchers, individuals who ate medium-chain triglycerides consume about 256 fewer calories a day.

Popcorn

No, not the popcorn you used to buy at the cinemas. That stuff is very unhealthy. We are talking about the one you can make at home in a pot or air-popper machine. A small amount of fat has a lot of calories, so you want to avoid commercially sold popcorn.

Popcorn is a whole grain food that is rich in fiber. Just 112 grams of it has 16 grams of fiber, meaning that it is quite filling. Some studies found that popcorn is more filling than many other popular snacks like potato chips or chocolates. So, if you do not have access to almonds for some reason, popcorn is a good alternative. Popcorn is very filling as it is rich in fiber and has a low energy density.

Water

People often say that drinking water helps with weight loss, and that is true. Drinking water boosts your metabolism by 24 to 30% over 1 to 1.5 hours, allowing you to burn a few more calories. In addition to drinking water frequently, you can also drink water before meals, as a study showed that drinking only half a liter of water about half an hour before meals help dieters consume fewer calories and lose about 45% more weight, compared to those who don't.

Eggs

Whole eggs have many health benefits, including weight loss. Studies show that when you replace a grain-based breakfast with eggs, it helps you eat fewer calories for the next 36 hours in addition to losing more weight and body fat. If you do not eat eggs, that is fine. You can get the same effect by consuming any high-protein food for breakfast.

Coffee

Have you ever noticed that, after drinking coffee, your hunger seems to just fade away? Coffee has been demonized unfairly. In fact, quality coffee is full of antioxidants and can have many health benefits. Many studies have shown that the caffeine in coffee can boost your metabolism by 3 to 11% and increasefat burning rate by up to 10 to 29%.

It is recommended that you drink black coffee as it is low in calories. Also, make sure you do not add sugar or other high-calorie ingredients to your coffee. That will just negate any benefits.

Green Tea

Just like coffee, green tea has many health benefits, one of which is weight loss. While it has a small amount of caffeine, it is full of powerful antioxidants called catechins, which works with caffeine to enhance fat burning. While scientific evidence is mixed, many studies agree that green tea can help you lose weight all the same.

Added Sugar

Added sugar is probably one of the worst things to have in a modern diet. A lot of people consume way too much of this stuff. Numerous studies have shown that the consumption of sugar and high-fructose corn syrup is associated with an increased risk of obesity, and other conditions such as heart disease and type 2 diabetes. If you want to lose weight, cut back on added sugar. Of course, it is easier said than done. Before you buy anything, make sure to read the labels because even some "health foods" can be chock-full of sugar.

Sugary Drinks

While we are on the subject of sugar, avoid sugary drinks such as soda and fruit juice. Sugar alone is bad enough, but sugar in its liquid form is even worse. Some studies show that calories from liquid sugar might be the leading cause of fat increase in the modern diet. For instance, a study shows that sugar-sweetened beverages are linked to a 60% increased risk of obesity in children for each daily serving. Here, it is worth mentioning that this also applies to fruit juice as well. While it tastes like fruit, it actually contains almost the same amount of sugar as any other soft drink like Coke.

Also, "diet" soda and other "zero calorie" drinks do not work as they are advertised. They certainly contain calories. Most importantly, they have sugar in them. If you drink these and take a test with your glucose meter, you will see the difference. They have effects, but not good ones. So, avoid them.

So, if you want something sweet in your mouth, eat whole fruit instead as it's a lot healthier. If you can't, then at least try to minimize the number of sugary drinks you drink.

Refined Carbs

Just like added sugar, you should also avoid refined carbs like the plague because refined carbohydrates have sugar and grains that have been stripped of their nutritious, fibrous arts. This includes white bread and pasta.

Studies have shown that refined carbs can cause a major spike in blood sugar, leading to hunger, cravings, and increased food intake a few hours later. Many cases of obesity are linked to the consumption of refined carbs. If you do wish to consume carbs, make sure to eat them with their natural fiber.

Low-Carb Diet

If you wish to get all the benefits of carb restriction, perhaps you should go all the way and commit to a low-carb diet. Many studies have shown that such a regimen can help you shed twice or even thrice as much weight as a standard low-fat diet while also improving your health.

Smaller Plates

Sometimes, you can trick your brain into thinking that you are eating the same amount of food when you are actually eating less by using smaller plates. You may be used to portioning your food based on how it fills your plate, so this trick may work for you. This has been shown to help some people eat fewer calories without realizing it. However, this does not affect everyone. The most noticeable effect is when this is done on overweight individuals.

Portion Control or Calorie Counting

Portion control, or basically eating less, or counting calories can be very useful for obvious reasons. Some studies have shown that keeping a food diary or taking pictures of your meals can help you lose weight.

In fact, anything that increases your awareness of what you are eating is most likely to be beneficial.

Keep Healthy Food Around

Instead of having snacks like chips laying around the home, tempting you every time you step into the room, why not replace them with healthy food? That way, when you become excessively hungry, you can snack on some healthy food instead. Your choice of snacks should be easily portable, and simple to prepare such as whole fruits, nuts, baby carrots, yogurt, and hard-boiled eggs.

Probiotic Supplements

Taking probiotic supplements that have bacteria of the Lactobacillus subfamily has been found to reduce fat mass in our body. However, this only applies to the lactobacillus subfamily, not the entire lactobacillus species. Some studies suggest that L. acidophilus actually causes weight gain.

Spicy Foods

Another trick you can use is by eating spicy food. For example, chili peppers contain capsaicin, which is a spicy compound that boosts metabolism and reduces your appetite slightly. However, that does not mean that you can lose a lot of weight just by eating spicy food over time because you may develop tolerance to the effect of capsaicin, which might limit its long-term effectiveness.

Aerobic Exercise

Another excellent way to burn calories and improve your physical and mental health is by doing aerobic exercise. It seems to be effective for losing belly fat, as the unhealthy fat tends to build up around your organs and cause metabolic disease.

Lift Weights

One of the worst side effects of dieting is that it often causes muscle loss and slows down metabolism, which reduces its effectiveness in terms of reducing fat weight. This slowdown and muscle lossare otherwise known as starvation mode.

One way to prevent this is by doing some resistance exercise such as lifting weights. Some studies have shown that lifting weights can help maintain a high level of metabolism and prevent you from losing muscle mass.

Of course, losing fat does not necessarily result in a toned body. You should also build up your muscles through resistance exercise.

Fiber

Fiber is often recommended for weight loss, although the evidence is mixed about this matter. Some studies show that fiber, especially viscous fiber, can increase satiety and help you control your weight for a long time.

Vegetables and Fruits

It should go without saying that eating vegetables and fruits is a lot healthier than fries and pizza. Vegetables and fruits have many properties that make them effective for weight loss because they contain a lot of fiber, but very few calories. They also have high water content, which means they have low energy density but are also very filling. As such, they prove to be very effective for weight loss, not to mention that they are very nutritious.

Chew Slower

It will take a while for your brain to register when you have eaten enough. If you eat quickly, then you would have already been overeating for quite a few bites already before your brain tells you that you have had enough. Some studies show that chewing slower helps you consume fewer calories and increases the production of hormones linked to weight loss. Moreover, you should also chew more thoroughly as that may reduce the calorie intake at a meal.

Sleep

Sleep is very underrated, and it may be the key to weight loss. Studies show that poor sleep is one of the biggest risk factors for obesity because it is linked to an 89% increased risk of obesity in children and 55% in adults.

Overcome Your Food Addiction

A recent study conducted on Americans and Europeans found that roughly 20% of them fulfill the criteria for food addiction. If you have food cravings and cannot seem to cut down on your eating no matter how hard you try, you may be a victim of food addiction. If that is you, then you should seek professional help as trying to lose weight without first overcoming food addiction is near impossible.

Protein

Protein is one of the most important constants in your weight loss equation. Having a diet mainly comprised of protein has been shown to boost metabolism by 80 to 100 calories a day while cutting off roughly 440 calories a day off your diet. A study shows that by having protein as a source of 25% of your total calorie intake, it reduces obsessive thoughts about food by 60% while also reducing the desire for late-night snacking in half. So, adding protein into your diet is a clever way to lose weight.

Whey Protein

While we are on the subject of protein, if you have problems getting it into your diet, consider taking a supplement, such as protein powder. A study shows that replacing some of your calories with whey protein can cause weight loss of about 8 pounds over time while also increasing your muscle mass.

Whole, Single-Ingredient Foods

More commonly known as real food, you can become leaner and healthier if you do yourself a favor and eat whole, single-ingredient foods. They are filling by nature, so it is very hard to gain weight if you base your diet on them.

Eat Healthily

Sometimes, diets may not work in the long term for you. We have already established that the same diet plan will have different effects on different people. Some studies show that dieting may lead to future weight gain. Instead of following a diet regimen, maybe you should just eat healthily. Aim to become healthier, happier, and fitter. It may be more effective for you to focus on nourishing your body instead of depriving it. Weight loss should come to you naturally then.

Chapter 7: Supercharging Your Weight Loss

Throughout the book, we have mentioned that intermittent fasting can help you get into ketosis, a body mode which burns fat much more effectively. You may be wondering if you can combine keto diets with intermittent fasting. The thing is, you certainly can.

Intermittent fasting is tricky when you are not on a ketogenic diet and the ketogenic diet gets a boost because your body goes into ketosis much faster if you fast.

Putting It into Practice

If you wish to raise your ketone levels or start your ketogenic journey along with your intermittent fasting one, you can try out this 3-day "fasting" protocol first and see if it works. We recommend that you start on a weekend as you would be resting by then. If things go awry, you know that you can just take a break for the rest of the weekend to let your body reset.

Start your 3-day trial on a Thursday evening, eat a ketogenic dinner and make that the last meal of the day. Sleep as you normally would.

Then, on Friday morning, start your day by walking within 30 minutes of waking up. If you need to, drink coffee or tea. However, limit your caffeine intake because you will excrete more minerals and fluid than usual. Have at least 1 liter of water with some added unrefined salt. Take a sip now and again as you walk to avoid cramping. Walk for a few hours and take a sip as needed. To make your walking hours productive, you can make phone calls or something similar. The idea here is to get you to use up your glycogen stores, which forces your body into deep ketosis. The faster you get into ketosis, the less time you will spend feeling drained. After walking, consume MCT oil a few times throughout the day because this gives you energy until your ketone levels elevate normally.

On Saturday morning, test your blood ketones by using a ketone blood testing kit. Your blood ketones should be at 0.7mmol or more. If you are at 0.7mmol, continue with your fast. If you are below that, consider walking for a few more hours and then retest.

For Saturday and Sunday day, add more MCT oil or coconut oil if you need a boost. You no longer need them when you are in deep ketosis. Also, incorporate some salts in your water throughout the day. This can be table salts or other electrolyte replacement pills.

At the end of Sunday, break your fast with a ketogenic meal.

Chapter 8: How to Stay Motivated

No diet and no fasting method is really easy and even intermittent fasting needs a bit of willpower, albeit a little and only at the start. There are, of course, ways to smoothen things up at the beginning so you can get over the hurdle at the start and feel right at home all throughout the fasting regime. Therefore, we have summarized a few tips here, so you can easily start the new diet.

For instance, it is very easy to get started with intermittent fasting using the 16:8 method. It may still be a bit hard to not eat for 16 hours at all. In this case, one should approach the implementation of the fast slowly. The beginning is a change in the diet from fast food and mostly heavy dishes to light and healthy dishes.

A healthy diet, especially at the beginning, should not have bread, with the exception of wholemeal bread. You should be introducing healthy food into your diet after every fasting period. So you can still eat your usual food within the meal times, but during the fasting, you may eat salad or raw food. As a result, the body gets used to it. This makes it much easier to get used to the real fast later on. At the start, you just set a meal that is the easiest for you. After a few weeks or months, you transition to another kind of meal. Then the next and in the end, you eat only lightly. Then you can start with the right fasting phase in the next step.

The fasting phase can be kept as-is at the beginning. As always, you can have your breakfast, lunch, snack, and dinner, which has now been converted to healthy stuff. Then, in the next step, you start to bring your dinner forward or, alternatively, to move the breakfast backward. No matter if you have decided on dinner or breakfast, you only move it by half an hour in one step. After a while, you approach it with another meal.

Those who have decided to have dinner will soon reach the time when there is no longer enough time between afternoon snack and dinner. Then it's time to merge the two together, creating a meal time to replace the snack time altogether. If you decided to have breakfast, it will eventually reach the point when it is too close to lunchtime. Then you cancel the breakfast and move the lunch a bit by moving lunchtime back slowly in 30-minute increments until it overlaps breakfast time and then shifts it to its original time.

Moreover, you can make the beginning of fasting easier by preparing mentally for it. It is important to know that pessimism is not a motivation. So if you accept starvation as motivation, there is no motivation to be found. You will, therefore, have no willpower to endure this. So, if you decided on trying out intermittent fasting, you need to have at least one important reason. Some people try it out because they are overweight, have health problems, or for any other reason. You need to know about this. The more you know, the more meaning it has and the more it motivates you. Then you can also withstand the hunger phases and avoid a relapse.

At the same time, you always have to bring positive thoughts. You should not think about hunger, but about yourhealth, you are trying to improve. One should not say that they are weak without food, but the body has time to regenerate and to be stronger.

The 16:8 method is easiest for the body and the easiest to integrate into your daily routine. Therefore, you should actually work with your diet and slowly transition into this regime. Especially as a beginner, the 16-hour fast seems to be very long, but here's the thing: you can skip half of it by sleeping for eight hours. You do not eat anything while your sleep anyway, so you are already making big progress when you sleep.

Furthermore, you should not make a big deal out of fasting. It is mainly about the time of sleep. For the meal times, you move them around only a bit to better suit your schedule. The whole thing is so simple and therefore requires neither great effort nor does it pose an insurmountable obstacle. So you are not putting yourself through a lot to get results.

When using the 16:8 method, you should not expect too much in a short time. Intermittent fasting and especially the 16:8 method aims at a slow and sustained weight loss. So if you try the scales, you will quickly notice that you only lose one to two kilos per month. But that's no problem because weight loss is progressing steadily without any implications.

If you also exercise while fasting, you may even find you gain weight under certain circumstances. This is because muscle cells are a lot heavier than fat cells. So, if you build muscles while losing fat simultaneously, you may either see little changes in weight or you may even gain weight. There is no need to be disheartened about this. The goal is to eliminate the fat in your body, which does not necessarily mean losing weight. Of course, it is important to see the progress in order to be motivated. But now we have just realized that you do not lose weight fast and, as you exercise, may even put on more weight. So how should youmeasure your success?

Success comes in two identifiable ways. The first is that you feel better and lighter. The body is not so much burdened by the toxins and regenerates over time. Accordingly, you feel energetic, fresh, and healthy. The second way also does not require a scale. You may not see your progress when you step on the scale and see the numbers, but you can feel the difference when you tighten your belt, put on your trousers, shirts, or when you buy new clothes, you may feel that you fit into them a lot easier. This is also more important than the kilosbecause after all, you do not want to lose them to be lighter, but to be slimmer, and that can be achieved very easily.

Fasting as a Lifestyle

Intermittent fasting is more than a diet. You can maintain it over long periods of time. Then, you will be slim and stay that way. So, you would feel better for longer than a moment. You will continue to feel better for a very long time. You can achieve a consistentresult if you stick to these pointers to help you incorporate fasting seamlessly into your lifestyle.

Start Slowly

First of all, take your time getting into fasting. It is not a diet, nor it is for a short time, nor it is to shed a few kilos. It is more of a marathon than a sprint. It is all about continuing eating normally over time, while slowly and steadily losing weight and improving your health.

So, start fasting slowly and give yourself time to get used to it. It generally takes two weeks for your body to get fully accustomed to a fasting regimen. So, do not just forgo meals in the name of getting slimmer. If you have problems getting used to a fasting regimen, we suggest you move two meals slowly together, e.g. moving breakfast forward in time and lunch backward in time, until the two overlaps. Then, move that meal time to a time that works best for you.

Of course, there is no need to adhere strictly to your eating time. If you have an appointment or a meeting, you can break out of your rhythm and plan for the next fasting period. Still, you should not constantly change the rhythms. Your body needs to adjust, and if you keep changing, it is the same as not having a consistent sleeping pattern. You will have your meal or enough sleep, but you will feel horrible every time.

Take Your Time

Most importantly, do not expect nor force rapid weight loss. Intermittent fasting is not a quick solution to weight loss. In fact, any quick fix solutions are most likely bad ones. Again, the whole thing is a marathon. It's about a steady, slow weight loss. This is also much healthier for the body.

By the way, if you are doing sports at the same time, you may not even see any change in weight. That's because you build muscle cells and they are much heavier than fat cells. If you want to see your success, look at your clothes. You might notice that they are looser than before.

Never exaggerate

We have talked about a few intermittent fasting methods and the OMAD method is one of the harder variants out there. We have also mentioned that you should experiment and find out which pattern works best for you. However, by "working best for you", we do not mean the method that yields the best results for you. The worst thing you can do to your body is overextending, trying to force a result, which is unsustainable and would often damage your health instead. Listen to your body. Try one of the three methods we discussed. Stick to a routine only if your body feels okay with. Do not force anything, because you'll only be frustrated and you'll destroy your motivation in the end.

Sleep

In the beginning, intermittent fasting is difficult. It is therefore important to always combine it with sleep as it will only bring you the least hunger. So you can then get started from there and don't have to spend too much time going on an empty stomach. Moreover, you should get more sleep than you normally would, especially if you attempt to fast for 24 to 72 hours or more. That way, you would wake up with more energy to spare.

Keeping Busy

You may find that you are thinking about food when you fast, especially at the beginning. This is common among beginners and veterans alike. There is a workaround, though. You can try to shift your focus and energy elsewhere. You can focus on the work you should be doing, an action movie you are dying to watch, or a lovely date with your partner. Do what you like so you will not notice that you are hungry. Oh, and if you go to the movies or go out with a partner, leave the eating activity out of the plan.

Sports

Sport is a nice help, but not a must. However, if you can, you should invest your new time and money in a little physical exercise. With it, you can build some muscle, and you also increase your performance. You also tighten your body and look better and younger. In addition, sport makes sure that you can reduce your daily stress and get better sleep. We will discuss sports and intermittent fasting in details in a later chapter.

Drinks enough and the right one

If you make intermittent fasting a part of your lifestyle, be sure to combine it with enough drinking. Detoxification does not work if you do not absorb water. In addition, enough fluid intake also prevents other ailments and illnesses. Basically, water is the simplest, cheapest and most effective medicine. Do not waste this opportunity for you and your body.

Find like-minded people

A hobby, occupation or lifestyle is so much more interesting if you can share it with someone. So, turn to the internet and share what you are doing. Find forums and exchange ideas. Convince your partner and your friends. Anything, when done by a group of people, is a hundred times more fun. Moreover, people around you also have great ideas, and it is fun to try them out together. After all, we feel the happiest when we have social interaction. The lack thereof creates dissatisfaction, which leads to overeating and obesity. So, be in touch with other people who fast intermittently like you. Facebook, Instagram, Reddit, and many other platforms out there host such a community that you can get into for free.

11 Tips to Make Fasting a Breeze

In this section, we will discuss the things you can do to make fasting more enjoyable for you.

Look Forward to It

It sounds strange as fasting can seem scary when you first start out. However, after a while, you may even enjoy it. After eating, strive toward the clarity, organization,and focus that comes with fasting. Focus on the fact that you do not need to think too much about food.

Put Off Until Tomorrow

Okay, procrastination is bad, but you can use it to your advantage. If you have a craving, tell yourself that you can enjoy it tomorrow. Most of the time, that craving will pass before tomorrow comes. It helps ease your mind when it knows that you will address it at a specific time later.

Wonder if You've Lost Weight

This does not mean forcing yourself to get on the scale as the number it spits at you does not tell the whole story. Instead, focus on how loose your clothes feel compared to how tight they were when you first started out fasting intermittently.

Consider Breaking the Fast

Everyone, even fasting veterans, sometimes think of this during their fasting period. Sometimes, your hunger gets the better of you or you feel left out when everyone else is enjoying their delicious meals. Many people consider breaking their fast a few times throughout the day. These thoughts are entirely normal, though self-sabotaging, it may help to entertain those thoughts for a while. There is no point in pretending that fasting is effortless. It does take some amount of willpower to get through it. IF will get easier, but pretending that it is a breeze is boring. So, entertaining the thought of smashing down a pizza may help make your fasting easier.

Sleep Early and Well

If you fast for long periods of time (24 to 72 hours), you may want the day to end fast so you can start eating again. This gets to you the most toward the end of your fasting period. When this happens, it is recommended that you sleep early. After all, you will most likely feel tired throughout your fasting days. You need to sleep to allow your body to rest so you can wake up feeling fresh the next day.

Chew Gum

When you are fasting, your body goes into ketosis easier, or the "fat burning mode" that produces ketones. Ketones may make you feel a bit fuzzy and give you bad breath. This can make those who fast very conscious whenever they open their mouths. To counter this, have some sugar-free gum handy and pop a piece when you are heading out or when you attend a meeting. That way, the gum can help cut down on the bad breath somewhat. Plus, gum is also helpful in preventing food cravings.

Have Some Coffee

Toward the end of the book, we will tell you more about how to drink coffee strategically. However, the idea is that your body is more sensitive to caffeine and its effect when you are in your fasted state. That way, you can capitalize on your body's sensitivity by drinking coffee as you would feel more energetic and your hunger better suppressed compared to when you drink it in your eating window.

Makeup

Sometimes, ladies just need to doll up a bit during their fasting days. You just need enough to make you feel empowered to push through the fasting days. It doesn't have to be strictly makeup, though. It can be clothing or whatever makes you feel better to get through the day.

Things like skinny clothing may help as well because you can feel the difference in how loose it feels now compared to before you started fasting. Plus, you can get to see just how slim your body has become after fasting for a long time.

All of this helps motivate you to keep fasting further.

Treats

Saving 80 to 100 calories of snack for the fasting day is a good idea, especially if you are just starting out, a woman, or fasting for long periods of time (24 to 72 hours). Having some healthy snacks ready helps get you through the fasting day as it can help fuel your body just enough without nullifying the calorie deficit you create. Plus, you may feel more secure when you fast because you know that you have some emergency fuel handy should you need it.

Drink Water

As mentioned at the beginning of the book, your body needs water to help detoxify itself. Moreover, a third of your body's water intake comes from the food you eat. Because you do not eat, you will need to get your fill of water elsewhere. So, drink more water during your fasting days. If you are thirsty, it is a sign that you are already dehydrated. Drinking plenty of water, more than you usually would, during your fasting day helps immensely.

Chapter 9: Women and Fasting

This section will cover some of the things that women need to know when they start fasting, particularly the complications they will face, how to deal with them, as well as other practical tips to make the entire experience more enjoyable for them. Women are expected to manage almost everything and excel at doing so. Frankly, it is outright impossible unless they have 48 hours a day to do everything. Alas, that is not the case, and we all live our lives in a constant rush, always under pressure and hardly have any time to relax. Women also have to deal with "that time of the month" that just makes their day all the more dreadful.

Is it Suitable for Women?

Because intermittent fasting has become more and more popular in recent years, many people have many questions. Its popularity is thanks to the fact that intermittent fasting does not tell you what to eat, unlike most diets. It instead focuses more on when you should eat by incorporating regular short-term fasts into your routine.

So, you can consume fewer calories, lose weight, and lower your risk of heart disease, diabetes, and other diseases altogether, all in your own convenience. However, some studies have suggested that intermittent fasting may not be equally beneficial for women like that to men. Again, it all boils down to how women's bodies function. So, women need to use a different approach to fasting to get the most out of intermittent fasting.

A study showed that blood sugar control worsened in women after fasting intermittently for three weeks, which is not the case for men. Some women even experienced changes to their menstrual cycles after they started fasting intermittently, which is not ideal for women. This unpleasant change is linked to the extreme sensitivity to calorie restriction in the female body. When calorie intake is low, a part of the brain called the hypothalamus is affected, which is the part that is responsible for hormone release.

Here, the lack of calorie intake disrupts the secretion of a hormone called gonadotropin, which helps release two reproductive hormones: luteinizing hormone and follicle stimulating hormone. Irregular periods, infertility, poor bone health, and other health effects result from the lack of communication between these two hormones and the ovaries.

While there are no comparable human studies, research on rats have shown that alternate-day fasting over 3 to 6 months caused a reduction in ovary size and irregular reproductive cycles in female rats. As such, it is recommended that women should try out a modified approach to intermittent fastings, such as a shorter fasting phase and fewer fasting days.

The Advantages of Fasting for Women

Fasting for women also carries the combined positive effects of crash diets, therapeutic fasting, and alkaline fasting. The downside is that it can take a while for it to be effective, especially if you are a woman. Still, the effects are there and they are sustainable, not to mention natural and healthy for your body. In addition, intermittent fasting offers us a lot of benefits, especially for us women. Let's have a look at them in detail.

The Meals

Women, in particular, are affected by every kind of diet change, as it is still them who often cook. So as soon as they want to eat something else or go on a diet, the burden of the change lies with them.

Intermittent fasting takes that problem away by allowing you to shop and prepare food as usual. You like soups, well, eat your soups. You love fries, then go ahead. You fancy a decent steak; there's nothing stopping you. Everything you eat so far, you continue to eat as usual. The change does not require you to start immediately reducing the amount of food you prepare. That comes with time by itself. So you cook everything as usual. But you can only miss a meal, but we'll get to that later. But that means you buy less and are at the store less often.

A study found that young men ate up to 650 fewer calories a day when they only had 4 hours to eat for the day. Another study on 24 healthy men and women utilized a longer, 36-hour fast on eating habits. While subjects did consume extra calories after the fasting day, their total calorie balance dropped by 1,900, which is a significant reduction.

A Better Sense of Well-Being

You can get the same detoxifying effect in the body by fasting intermittently, just like men. You will feel better and stronger as your body works to flush the toxins out of your body slowly and steadily. With that, you can do something again and enjoy life. More than that, your organs also perform better, making life more enjoyable.

Your Skin Gets Better

This is considered to be a huge plus for women. You understand what it is like to look young again, with a tight, healthy, and wrinkle-free skin. Intermittent fasting takes away the excessive acid out of the body, allowing the connective tissues to become firmer and more flexible again. This tightens the skin, making it shine and look younger with fewer wrinkles.

This acid also causes your skin to look unpleasant. Scales and lichens are often caused by this acid, which also creates a perfect environment for fungi and bacteria that lead to infection and dandruff. Here, intermittent fasting allows the body to flush out the acid. Then, the skin changes to allow the natural protective film on your skin to regenerate. Fungi and bacteria will find it harder to thrive as there is greater resistance. This translates to no more scales, lichens, and pimples.

Your Nails and Hair Get Better

This acid also affects the nails and hair. They can regenerate to have that youthful appearance again as soon as the acid leaves the body. Your nails will be nice and shiny as your hair gains in volume and shine. Intermittent fasting thus acts like a total rejuvenation on your body.

The Fat on the Stomach Disappears

The idea behind intermittent fasting is to create a calorie deficit from the food you eat, forcing the body to feed on the fat instead. That way, you will break down your fat in your stomach and everywhere in your body slowly and steadily. Of course, you should not expect a miracle. You will not lose 5 kilos a day or a week, but it is about one to three kilos a month. However, since this is done steadily and a year has 12 months, you can easily figure out when you will have reached your desired weight.

Better Mood

Many women know that food dictates their mood. The food is supposed to give us energy. Most of the time though, women tend to cook for themselves so the idea of eating becomes stressful instead. It pollutes your body and thus your mind, but it also has a direct effect on your mood. Now, if you take a break by not eating, therefore taking away the stress of cooking, you'll soon feel lighter and happier again. Last but not least, intermittent fasting also relieves your digestion, giving you more energy. More energy means a better sense of well-being, therefore, a better mood.

A Better Sleep

Eating too much ensures that the body does not rest properly. The result is a restless sleep that lacks the important deep sleep phase. You cannot relax and do not feel rested. But with intermittent fasting, this is a thing of the past. Eating less means that your body can switch off more easily and get a deeper sleep. When well-rested, you are better equipped to take on the next day.

Heart Health

Heart disease is one of the leading causes of death worldwide. Leading risk factors for the development of heart disease include high blood pressure, high LDL cholesterol and high triglyceride concentrations. A study on 16 obese men and women showed that intermittent fasting lowered blood pressure by 6% in eight weeks, not to mention lowered LDL cholesterol by 25%, and triglycerides by 32%.

However, this is only one study. There is a lack of connection between intermittent fasting and the decrease of LDL cholesterol and triglyceride levels, as well as a lack of consistency as to how much when the subjects are put through intermittent fasting. A study conducted on 40 normal-weight individuals found that during the four weeks of intermittent fasting during Ramadan it did not result in a reduction in LDL cholesterol or triglycerides.

So, we need higher-quality studies with more robust methods before researchers can fully understand the effect of intermittent fasting on heart health.

Diabetes

Intermittent fasting may also be useful in managing and reducing your risk of developing diabetes. Just like continuous calorie restriction, intermittent fasting seems to reduce some of the risk factors of diabetes by lowering insulin levels and reducing insulin resistance.

In a randomized controlled study with more than 100 overweight or obese women taking part in six months of intermittent fasting, it is reported that the insulin levels decreased by 29%, and insulin resistance reduced by 19%. Blood sugar levels, however, remained the same.

Another study conducted on pre-diabetic individuals over 8 to 12 weeks of intermittent fasting resulted in lowered insulin levels by 30% and blood sugar levels reduced by 5%. In terms of blood sugar levels, intermittent fasting may not be as beneficial for women compared to men.

A study found that blood sugar control actually worsened for women after 22 days of alternate-day fasting, while men experienced no drawbacks. Despite this side effect, the reduction in insulin and insulin resistance would still reduce the risk of diabetes, especially for women with pre-diabetes.

Weight Loss

As explained earlier, intermittent fasting can be an effective and simple way to shed some weight over long periods of time, making it very sustainable. You can do it as regular short-term fasts and you will still be able to shed a few pounds. Many studies suggest that intermittent fasting is as effective as calorie-restricted diets for short-term weight loss.

A 2018 review of studies on overweight adults found that intermittent fasting led to an average weight loss of 6.8kg over 3 to 12 months. Another review found that intermittent fasting reduced body weight by 3 to 8% in overweight or obese individuals in over 3 to 24 weeks. Moreover, its participants reported that their waist circumference decreased by 3 to 7% over the same amount of time.

It is also worth pointing out that the long-term effects of intermittent fasting for women remain to be seen. In the short term, though, intermittent fasting seems to help in losing weight. However, how much you lose will most likely depend on how many calories you consume when you are not fasting, and how long you follow this fasting lifestyle.

Other Health Benefits

A number of studies on animals and humans suggest that intermittent fasting may yield other health benefits such as:

- Preserve muscle mass: Intermittent fasting seems to be effective at retaining muscle mass, which helps you burn more calories even when you are resting.
- Increased longevity: Intermittent fasting has been shown to extend lifespan in mice and rats by 33 to 83%, but such an effect is not confirmed in humans.
- Improved psychological well-being: A study found that eight weeks of intermittent fasting decreased depression and binge eating while improving body image in obese individuals.
- Reduced inflammation: Some studies show that intermittent fasting can minimize key markers of inflammation, which is a big deal as chronic inflammation can lead to weight gain and many other health problems.

Best Types of Fasting Methods for Women

As always, you need to find the right fasting regimen for you because there is no one-size fits all approach here even for women. As a woman, you should take a modified approach to intermittent fasting so as not to mess up your hormones and make yourself feel horrible. That means shorter fasting periods, less frequent eating or consuming a small number of calories in the fasting phase. Here are some variations of the fasting methods we have discussed:

- The 16:8 method: Instead of starting fasting for 16 hours a day and eating within 8 hours, you should start with 14-hour fasts and work your way up to 16 hours.
- Crescendo Method: You can fast between 12 to 16 hours twice or thrice a week. Fasting days should not be consecutive and they should be spaced evenly across the week.
- OMAD method: Start by fasting for 14 to 16 hours a day just like the 16:8 method first, then work your way up to a 24-hour fast. Again, only do this once or twice a week.
- You fast every other day, but you eat normally on your non-fasting days. That means 20 to 25% of your usual calorie intake, which is about 500 calories, during the fasting days.
- The 5:2 diet: Also known as the fast diet, you restrict your calorie intake to 25% (roughly 500 calories), and fast for two days a week, and eat normally the other five days. Allow one day between fasting days to allow the body to rest.

Whichever you choose, it is crucial that you eat well during non-fasting periods. So, healthy food is the way to go as eating unhealthy, calorie-dense food will only counteract the effect fasting has on your body. Whatever you do, it is best to consult your doctor before you start, and listen to your body. Only follow a fasting regimen that you can tolerate and sustain in the long-term that does not result in any negative health consequences.

Getting Started

So, where do you start as a woman? It is simple. In reality, chances are that you have actually fasted before. Many people skip breakfast or dinner, therefore following one of the fasting methods we have previously discussed. So, just pick one of them and start doing it. See what works for you. However, we recommend that you start with the Crescendo method as it is the friendliest to women and beginners alike. Then, move on to the 16:8, 5:2, alternate-day fasting, then OMAD method as the difficulty scales smoothly. We suggest that you follow each method for about two weeks so your body has time to adjust, then work your way up.

However, you do not necessarily need to follow this plan. An alternative is to fast whenever it suits you. You can skip meals from time to time when you do not feel hungry, or when you do not have time to cook. At the end of the day, what matters is finding a method that works best for you and your lifestyle, not which fasting method you choose.

Safety and Side Effects

Again, we do not recommend women following the original variation of any fasting regimen as it can be too much for their bodies to handle and create many health complications down the road.

That being said, some studies have reported that fasting may introduce certain side effects such as hunger, mood swings, lack of concentration, reduced energy, headaches, and bad breath on fasting days. There are plenty of stories out there of women who said that their menstrual cycle stopped while following an intermittent fasting diet, most likely a result from the lack of interaction of certain hormones with their ovaries, which we have mentioned previously. If you have a medical condition, you should also consult with your doctor before trying out intermittent fasting.

Women should consult doctors if they:

- Have fertility problems or a history of amenorrhea (missed periods)
- Are pregnant, breastfeeding, or trying to conceive
- Are underweight, malnourished, or have nutritional deficiencies
- Have diabetes, or regularly experience low blood sugar levels
- Have a history of eating disorders

As we mentioned time and time again, everybody varies. Most of the time, you will do just fine. However, if you ever notice or experience any problems, such as loss of your menstrual cycle, you must stop immediately.

Chapter 10: Exercise and Fasting

You can maximize your weight loss process by exercising, which can be done easily considering that intermittent fasting is easy to follow. This will bring stunningly better outcomes. Be that as it may, it has its own issues. Therefore, you need to know which sport you should do and how you should do it.

Why Sports?

Our body is still prepared to confront hardships. It expects hardship. Actually, we have never been any more secure. We live in comfort and abundance, and there is no compelling reason to spend a great deal of physical strength to sustain ourselves. Because of that, our body keeps accumulating energy it expects to be used one day, which never comes. Subsequently, we put on a little weight each day. That is the reason why practicing is vital. When this occurs, we will live much healthier and feel better.

Without exercise, the body, the muscles specifically, is not used or strained. Over time, your muscles will be weak, and you will eventually rue the day that you skippedexercising. Now, even if we don't exercise, our muscles will still be strong enough to allow us to walk around and do our tasks because we at least have trained them that much. That may be enough in most situations, but that's about all. What is the result? As soon as we push ourselves a little bit more, it will be too much. Worse still, when we spend a third of the day at work and come home, we feel tired and beaten and can do nothing more. The muscles will only be capable enough to do just enough work that you need to be done for the day. Do we really want that? For me, not really. Of course, we, especially women, need to do more than the bare minimum to get anywhere in life. That means cooking a delicious meal for the weekend, get that report done before the deadline, or attend a party. For that, my body should be able to handle a little more stress sometimes.

If we don't do sports, at that point we don't expend the stress hormones that we develop throughout the day. This implies our body can't rest completely and we can't unwind.

If we do not do sports, the body hardly sees a difference between day and night. This is because we spend most of the day depleting the mental energy, and not physical energy. So, even though we are mentally tired, the body is still quite energetic. This means we can hardly rest and get enough sleep and, above all, worsen our sleep quality causing us to wake up feeling groggy.

Sport is so important in our lives. We make our bodies stronger so that we are better prepared for challenges and also for everyday life. Sport makes sure that we reduce stress makes us sleep better.

Intermittent fasting helps to detoxify our bodies. Sport, together with intermittent fasting, improves our health considerably. This is not least due to the fact that sport gets our circulation going, which is conducive to detoxification.

Sport together with intermittent fasting accelerates weight loss. But we do not just lose the body fat faster, we replace it with muscle and, while the scale does not show you that, you will look better.

Speaking of better forms, sport is also a means to correct aesthetics. We just look better, because the right muscles in the right places also bring out our shape better. At the same time, our skin becomes firmer and our wrinkles less visible.

Another thing you need to know is that muscle cells always burn fat even when we do not use them when we exercise. That means those who train an hour a day to build muscle is basically burning fat 24 hours a day.

What Exercise Should I Try Out?

Just like intermittent fasting, you will need to find the one that works for you. Of course, the main idea here is to help you lose weight, not gain bulky muscles. So, lifting weights is out of the question unless you want to build muscles. If you are young, a whole-body workout is probably the best for you. If you are old, you should go for everyday sports.

A total body workout consists of various endurance and muscle exercises. The idea here is to build the muscles evenly throughout the body. Of course, there is no need to go overboard and achieve Arnold's level of muscles here. We speak of some weights for the right muscle groups. Your legs, hips,and stomach will be well-formed and firm. Even your chest will look great.

Everydayexercise should also combine endurance and muscle training. But there should be variations, ranging from very easy to difficult. Let's start with the easy part. If you are not so young, you should go for a walk. This brings a lot of fresh air into the lungs, as the whole body moves. At the same time, it builds a little muscle, but not too much that you have to worry. The most important thing here is to get the circulation going and strengthen it.

If you are young, you can walk at a brisk pace and with a weight of one or two kilos in each hand. This will also get the circulation going and get a bigger impact on the muscles. If you are in the early stage of adolescence or really young, try going for a walk by jogging with the dumbbells in your hand. You get to actively work all of your muscles and consume a lot of calories. Above all, we will pump so much oxygen through our bodies that we feel young and fresh even hours after the exercise.

You can also cycle as an alternative as it also engages all the muscles in your body. The circulation gets going as you pedal and it is also a great way to train your leg muscles. You will also engage all other muscles by trying to steer and balance the bike as you go.

The best option, however, is swimming. Here the circulation and every single muscle in the body is stressed. At the same time, the joints are spared from the strain. This will make everyone fast and slim, without fear of damage.

What Should a Training Session Look Like?

A training session consists of the warm-up, the actual training, and the transition phase. It's easy for everyday training. At the start, you swim in a relaxed manner or cycle slowly. That way, your breathing and heart rhythm can get up to pace to prepare the body for actual stress. This phase should be between 10 to 15 minutes long.

The next phase is the actual training. Here we run, swim and ride the bike in our real training pace. Here we should be careful to choose a pace at which we are still comfortable. We should not feel dizzy or hyperventilate. This phase lasts about 30 minutes.

The cooldown phase is the end and should slow down the body, allowing it to relax. You should feel your body slow down, and returning to a relaxed state during the transition. Most notably, the heart rate and the breathing rate will slow down. This phase should be the same length as the warm-up, i.e. 10 to 15 minutes.

The whole body workout also works with weights. Here we couldjog or bike as a warmup or cooldown, before and after we start using the dumbbells. The dumbbell training takes place in sets or intervals. Each set consists of 10 to 15 repetitions (reps) with the same dumbbell and the same movement without stopping. Again, you need to experiment and see which weight is right for you. If you can do more than 15 reps in one go, then you need to move on to a heavier weight. However, if you cannot make 10 in one go, return to lighter a weight. Of course, make sure your posture is proper throughout the training. Ten bad reps do not do your body as good as one good rep.

Each exercise should consist of 4 to 6 sets. Between the sets, there is a little break of one to two minutes. After each exercise, there is a break of 3 to 5 minutes.

Timing

It is also important to do sport at the right time and to ensure that it is properly timed throughout the week. Lighter everyday sports in the form of walking can be completed every day. All other sports need a firmer training regime.

It is just as important to exercise at the right time throughout the week. Casual, lighter everyday sports such as walking can be done every day whereas others need a firmer training regimen, especially those intended to build muscles as you need to work on different muscle groups each day.

During the exercise, we cause micro tears in our muscles, damaging them. This is all part of the process. You see, muscle growth is only possible if you cause tissue damage to them. That way, our muscles grow as they heal. The entire point of working out for muscle growth is to cause this injury. Then our body repairs the damage and makes the muscles stronger so that next time they can sustain more wear and tear. Nevertheless, we must keep this damage in mind and deal with it.

The first consequence of exercising is muscle injury, which does not permit everyday exercise for the same muscle group. There must be at least one rest day between training days so the muscles have time to regenerate. This allows us to work out three days a week, with one training day followed by one rest day.

What is also equally important is the right amount of training time. Here, a distinction should be made between the 16:8 and OMAD method. For the 16:8 method, exercises should be done so that the end of the workout coincides with the end of fasting. This has two advantages.

First, we have no fresh food in our body. This means that throughout our training, our body uses its fat reserves to meet its energy needs.

Second, after training, our body needs a lot of building materials to regenerate. But since our fasting has just ended with training, we can now feed these materials through the food.

Chapter 11:Other Practical Tips

In this chapter, we will discuss other tips you can incorporate into your fasting regimen to optimize your weight loss.

Common Fasting Mistakes

Fasting has been used for a while, but only a few really know about it. As a result, many people cannot get it right. This results in unsuccessful, unhealthy fasting, which would raise criticism against fasting as a whole. If you want your fasts to be effective, you need to avoid these five mistakes.

The first and most important mistake is not to obsess over the meticulous details. For intermittent fasting, all you need to do most of the time is skip breakfast. You only eat lunch and dinner, and you're good to go. Also, if you do decide to dig further into the matter, make sure you consult your doctor and do thorough research. The last thing you want to do to your body is put it through something that you do not really know about. As mentioned earlier, you may overeat. This is often aggravated by the idea that you fast and tend to try to compensate for the low-calorie intake the previous day.

Therefore, you would not reach the calorie deficit, and may instead build up a surplus in your body, causing it to become even fatter. So, if you want to get into fasting, do your due diligence and research thoroughly so you know what you want. As mentioned previously, consult your doctor before you attempt to fast because you may have certain medical technicality that prevents you from doing so, or make the experience a living hell. Moreover, you should have a general plan that includes a general idea of the nutritional value of food. Of course, you do not need to take out your calculator and start counting calories. But you should know a few things like pizza contains enough energy you need for the whole day and that a hamburger has multiple times the calories of a salad.

If you want to get it right, you need a plan and this plan must start from your current state, which is the time before you start fasting. What calorie quantity and nutrient distribution was there at that time? From there, you need to look at your calorie intake, how much you want and how do you want this to be distributed over the day. How much meat, how many fries, how many vegetables, and so on.

Another mistake that people often make is that, whether they have a plan or not, when they start fasting and finish their first fasting phase, they develop cravings. This often happens, but people often lose control when there are temptations right around the corner. They eat too much and they lose their progress. Intermittent fasting, for example, does not mean alternating between fasting and feasting. It means that fasting is followed by a meal phase, which is the time when you feed yourself normally before fasting again. Of course, the initial phase of food deprivation will lead to craving, but you need to do everything in your power to resist.

Intermittent fasting is one of the easiest diet regimes out therethat requires minimal willpower and perseverance compared to other diet methods. It is rather obvious from the start, but we want to stress how easy it is to maintain fasting intermittently. You just need to discipline yourself at the start because this is the period when you feel the most uncomfortable. It helps you to know that you will eat again very soon. However, just because it requires no effort does not mean that you can lower your guard. You need to maintain your fast during the fasting phase, and the subsequent fasting phases for this to work. Because fasting does not yield an immediate result, it may be disheartening to see that you have made little progress over the week. As mentioned earlier, fasting is a sustainable method of weight loss. You can just stick to your usual diet and fast to start losing weight.

There are two things that can be helpful here. First, plan properly as we mentioned. Having a plan makes it easier to stick to. Just make sure you stick to that plan. Another thing is that you should keep in mind that cravings will pass eventually. Once you have gone through some fasting phases, your body will get used to it and it just does not ask for more. Then you will be perfectly comfortable with your 8 hours daily fasting and no longer feel them cravings.

However, those who indulge in their cravings, do not just cancel the effect of the intermittent fasting immediately. It aggravates their situation because the cravings lead to a surplus amount of calories being consumed, which deposit themselves as fat, but also too many unhealthy foods will be consumed to satisfy their taste buds. This introduces toxins into the body and further damaging the body and reduce its performance. You really have to work the first few days on yourself and make sure that you eat normally after fasting.

The third mistake is just the opposite of the second mistake, which is the lack of food. This usually happens because you want to force results, instead of being patient and achieve a lasting effect. The body will respond by switching to starvation mode. This means it lowers metabolism rate to preserve energy. As a result, you do not have enough food for yourself and at the same time, you still do not lose weight. This can lead you into a vicious cycle, because you may reduce your food consumption even further in order to lose more weight. But then you will soon feel like people do in a crash diet. It is no longer comfortable and the body will start feeding on your muscles. If then the nutrition given is too low, it threatens the yo-yo effect, where it will store even more energy the next time you eat. Until then, however, you will feel limp, have no energy and be prone to depression.

The fourth mistake is too much coffee. Sure, you can still drink coffee during intermittent fasting. However, you should only drink it in moderation because it is addicting and it suppresses our appetite. The addiction makes us crave for more coffee and the appetite suppression makes us not feel hungry. This creates a vicious cycle. Coffee is not the problem and it actually inhibits the appetite, which makes you fast, especially in the morning, good. But if a cup is not enough for you, then the whole thing will be different. It gets really problematic when you drink up to three or four cups.

When you drink coffee during your fast, it gets into the blood much quicker and much more. The result is the release of adrenaline and cortisone. Both of them have an appetite-suppressing effect because these are the hormones that are supposed to make it possible to fight or flight, and hunger is an obstacle. At the same time, both hormones bring energy to the body. But they break up the sugar in the blood and the body gets the power that it needs for the fight or the flight. But the blood sugar level drops and what stays behind when the effect of the hormones has stopped is a craving for sweets. This then makes the fast even more difficult or ensures that sugar will be consumed in a large quantity for the next feeding phase.

The fifth mistake is the wrong organization and the wrong execution of meals. So, take it easy when you start fasting and eat the kind of food that your body can digest easily. It is recommended to eat something easy for the body, such as at breakfast. Most people, however, just skip breakfast but then eat something heavy for lunch. This then burdens the digestive system, which now consumes a lot of energy to break down the food. That also means that we have much less energy for our other tasks. We then feel tired and cannot do anything. A better alternative would be to eat something that the body can break down easily, even at noon.

The sixth mistake is to plan every single detail, without flexibility. It makes sense to have a plan, but it cannot anticipate or factor in all uncertainties. Here, you have to be flexible and able to react to the circumstances. So, for example, if you have to go on a business trip, are invited to an important party, or the daily routine is otherwise disrupted, you have to be able to react and adjust your planning. The important thing is that the exceptions really remain exceptions and the changes are not a habit.

Other Fasting Tips

In this section, we will look at other tips that do not quite fit in with the others. These are equally helpful and relatively easy to implement. They are:

Eating Window

The idea of fasting comes down to spending most of your conscious time in the fasted state. As you may have guessed, intermittent fasting is not a rigid regimen. Instead, it can be very flexible. It is not about some arbitrary eating window, but rather a personalized approach to eating within that window after you normally wake up. For instance, if you wake up by 5 am, you should have a meal around 10 am to 12 pm. Alternatively, if you wake up at 10 am, then your first meal should be around 3 to 5 pm.

4 to 7 hours is a perfect amount of time to spend in the fasted state day when you are conscious. Some people find that 6 hours is the most comfortable. However, you should listen to your body to determine when you should eat your first meal. Some people prefer to eat well into the day while others prefer eating four hours after rising. Find that perfect eating window and stick to it. However, keep in mind that it may change in the future, so your body is the only way to tell when you should shift the window.

Use Caffeine Strategically

If you do not drink coffee during your fasting period, then you probably should. You see, caffeine is stimulating you more when you ingest it in a fasted state. Plus, coffee can enhance the effects of fasting as it stimulates metabolism, suppresses appetite, gives you more energy, elevates fat mobilization as well as heightens alertness.

However, you should drink caffeine strategically. Its effects weaken the more you drink it, making it ineffective in suppressing appetite and boosting energy. Drink coffee during the fasting phase to maximize its effects. We recommend that you drink two cups of black coffee during the fasting phase and at no other point in the day. If you want to drink something hot during the day, drink tea instead. We understand that not everyone likes black coffee, but this is the purest caffeine you can drink. Eventually, you will develop a fondness for black coffee anyway.

Exercise Strategically

When you exercise during the fasting phase, you should base the former off low volume strength to build muscle and strength. If you only want to burn calories, low-intensity workouts like walking work the best. If you want to do some conditioning work, limit it to short interval sessions about 20 minutes long.

Unless you are a competitive athlete and need to do skill work for your sport, there is no need for more training. Drawn-out interval sessions or circuit routines or high volume workout sessions will cause you to burn much more energy, leaving you feeling very hungry during your fast not to mention that these forms of training are actually unnecessary in nature and only hampers your progress from your strength and muscle-building sessions.

So, keep your exercise at low volume strength instead. We recommend you focus on having fun during the workout rather than trying to inflict as much pain onto yourself as possible at the gym. Recreational sports such as yoga or martial arts are a great alternative to some form of extreme exercises such as CrossFit, p90x, andhour-long running sessions.

Intense training will only hamper your progress. Because intermittent fasting is a great tool for staying lean, we suggest making the most out of it by focusing your efforts on building strength and muscle. You can maybe add some light activity such as brisk walking now and again, and maybe do some short sprints if you want to.

Eat Fruit Strategically

As mentioned earlier, fruit (not fruit juice) is great as a snacking option if you feel hungry. It can make you feel full for longer and replenish your liver's glycogen. When it is depleted from long fasts, the liver sends a signal to the brain that triggers hunger.

You can tone down this hunger by eating some fruits if you feel hungry toward the end of your fasting phase. Plus, by replenishing your liver's glycogen, you help your body to shift back to an anabolic state.

So, when is the best time to grab this healthy snack? You should eat it when you have a relatively empty stomach, especially when the carbohydrate stores are low. This ensures that the carbs you consume goes directly to replenish the liver's glycogen store. This store is often topped off already if you had a big meal with carbs. More fruits after this will only lead to weight gain as the energy derived from the fruits will be stored as fat.

We recommend you have a few servings of fruit a day to ward off hunger before getting the rest of your carbs from potatoes and rice, which are rich in starches and better at restocking the muscle's glycogen. Here, we recommend you have an apple before lunch and dinner, and a banana occasionally before bed. Because bananas have high glucose content, they are a better option when it comes to replenishing muscle glycogen compared to most fruits. They also trigger our brain to release a hormone called serotonin, which helps us relax and improves sleep quality. Moreover, bananas are also a good source of magnesium and potassium, which promote muscle relaxation and further enhance your sleep quality.

Eat Big

Okay, not in the sense of making up for the calories lost. That defeats the purpose of intermittent fasting. If this is your first time trying out intermittent fasting, you may notice that you eat bigger meals compared to what you are used to. If you do not adjust your meals properly, you will have a very low-calorie intake and nutrients and hunger will be two of the most prominent problems in your endeavor. You may even feel tempted to snack on junk food to make up for the calories, which will destroy your progress entirely.

It is true that the entire idea of intermittent fasting is to create a calorie deficiency that leads to weight loss. However, that does not mean you should skimp on your meals because you put yourself at risk of becoming very hungry. Moreover, you want to include lots of protein within your meals to ensure that you get your protein number as well as to encourage satiety. So, it is okay to eat slightly larger meals throughout the day as long as the calorie deficit is still there.

Things will become so much easier when you feel full while still losing body fat. If you go too low in calories and eating just two normal meals a day, you put yourself at a massive calorie deficit and your fasts will be quite difficult. So, do not be scared of eating more than what initially seems reasonable.

Focus Elsewhere

Sometimes, to make fasting a breeze, you just need to forget the fact that you are fasting in the first place. This allows you to integrate fasting into your lifestyle very easily, soon youwill forget that you are doing this to lose weight and instead think of it as how you prefer to live every day. Intermittent fasting is supposed to be that extra add-on that many people overlook, but those who do use it geta great result.

However, there is no point in trying too hard to do it. Sticking to it is not that hard, and intermittent fasting is one of those things that you just leave there and let it run its course. You will be shocked by the result, but it will be one or two years away. If you stick to it, you will get results. Try not to force it and you will do just fine.

Common Weight Loss Mistakes

Losing weight can be difficult for many people as we do not lose the same amount of weight even if we follow the exact regimen. Sometimes, you may feel that you have followed everything to the letter, but still, do not get the results you were promised. When that happens, it is easy to become frustrated since you put yourself through everything for nothing. If that is you, perhaps you have made one of these common mistakes:

Focusing on the Scale Weight

The scale does not tell the whole story, as you have already guessed. You may be using the wrong tool to measure your progress. You may feel that you are not losing nearly enough weight despite the fact that you did your very best to follow the diet regimen. Just because the scale spits the same number at you as the last time does not mean that you are not losing weight. The scale is not accurate in telling you how much body fat you have lost. It only measures weight, which is actually comprised of many things such as fluid fluctuations and how much food is still in your system. Plus, you should also take muscle mass into consideration if you exercise regularly. You see, the idea of fasting is not to lose weight specifically. Rather, it focuses on reducing your body fat. In fact, your weight can fluctuate by about two kilos over the course of the day, depending on how much you eat and drink.

Things are even more complicated for women. You see, certain hormonal changes in women such as the increase in estrogen levels can lead to greater water retention, which also prevents them from losing weight.

Still, there are many factors that make the scale spit the same number. It does not matter what it says. There areother alternatives to tell how much body fat you have lost. You may already be losing fat weight in your body, but the number does not change simply because your body retains enough water to maintain the same number. Of course, there are plenty of things you can do to lose water weight, but that's not the point of intermittent fasting.

Moreover, if you have been working out, the muscle mass you accumulate throughout the workout routine may even outweigh the fat loss, which might give you the illusion that the fast or any diet regimen you have done is ineffective. A good way to tell if you are losing fat weight is when you put on your clothes. You may feel that they are looser, especially around the waist, even though you have a stable scale weight. Your waist circumference may go down, and you can measure that by using a tape measure, or take monthly pictures of yourself so you can compare how much fitter you have become since you have started.

Too Many or Too Few Calories

In Buddhism, Buddha taught humans to walk the middle path. In that context, it means to maintain a balance between pleasure and pain. Too much pain is torture. Too much pleasure is debauchery. The same can be said in the health and fitness world, any extreme is detrimental. While you need to create a calorie deficit to lose weight, it can be counterproductive as they can cause your body to go into its emergency starvation mode that slows down metabolism and may lead to muscle loss. Slower metabolism rate means your body spends less energy, meaning that you will have a calorie surplus next time you eat, which will lead to weight gain, not to mention that you may feel horrible. Studies show that very low-calorie diets less than 1,000 calories a day can lead to muscle loss and slow down metabolism significantly (NCBI: 19198647).

For many years, people believe that if your daily calorie intake is lower than 3,500 a week, you would lose about 0.5kg. However, more recent studies suggest that people lose weight differently because calorie deficit is different from person to person. So, a baseline to create a calorie deficit also varies. You might feel that you are not eating as many calories, but the reality is that we all tend to underestimate and underreport how much we eat.

According to a two-week study on ten obese people (NCBI: 1454084), subjects reported to consumed only 1,000 calories a day and the subsequent lab testing showed that they actually took in in about 2,000 calories a day. There are a few reasons why we underestimate the number of calories we eat, one of which is that we eat healthy food that ishigh in calories such as nuts and cheese. The key to controlling how much you eat is by watching your portion size.

Too Little or Too Much Exercising

It is normal to be losing muscle mass alongside fat mass during weight loss, although how much you lose them depends on various factors. If you do not exercise at all while fasting, you are prone to more muscle mass loss and a drop in your metabolic rate.

On the other hand, exercising might also help you minimize how much muscle mass you would lose while maximizing fat loss and prevent your metabolism from slowing down. The more lean mass you have, the easier it is for you to lose and continue to lose weight.

As we mentioned previously, to any extreme can be detrimental. Too much exercise can also cause problems. Some studies show that excessive exercise is not sustainable for many people in the long term, and may lead to stress (NCBI: 23404767, 26707388, 23667795). It might slow down your muscle gain progress, or grind it to a halt altogether. Plus, it may even slow the production of a hormone that regulates stress response called adrenal hormones. So, too much exercise is neither healthy or effective. Therefore, do not force your body to burn more calories through excessive exercising.

Instead of lifting excessively, feeling sore and drained at the end of your session so you can force your body to burn those extra calories, you should instead take it easy and lift weights or do cardio several times a week instead. That way, you establish a system of sustainable weight loss and maintain a relatively high metabolic rate.

Not Lifting Weights

While we are talking about exercising, you may not lose weight because you are not lifting enough weights. Weight lifting is a form of resistance exercise and is very crucial for weight loss. Lifting weight is one of the best ways to gain muscle and boost metabolic rate, not to mention improving overall body composition and boosting belly fat loss.

In fact, there was a review of 15 studies with over 700 people and they found that the best way to lose weight seems to be a combination of weightlifting and aerobic exercise (NBCI: 24358230).

Low-Fat or "Diet" Foods

Natural, whole foods are considered to be some of the healthiest things you can put into your digestive system. Because there is a growing health craze about weight loss, many companies exploit this need and put out processed low-fat foods or "diet" foods, which may not be as good as they sound. They are actually loaded with sugar so they taste better.

For instance, a cup of "low-fat", fruit-flavored yogurt has up to 47 grams of sugar, which is about 20% of the yogurt itself. So, instead of keeping you full, these low-fat products will instead put your hunger into overdrive, causing you to eat more as if eating that much sugar in such a small amount of food is not bad enough. So, instead of eating those foods, eat only the foods that are not processed, or as minimally processed as possible in combination with other nutritious foods.

Overestimate Calories Burned During Workout

Many people believe that exercising helps put their metabolism on overdrive. This is only partially true since exercises only increase metabolic rate slightly. It is actually very underwhelming. Studies show that both normal and obese people often overestimate how many calories they burn during exercise, often by a large amount. Another study had participants burn between 200 and 300 calories during exercise sessions. Subjects reported that they had burned more than 800 calories, and this led them to believe that they can eat more, which they did (NCBI: 21178922). Still, it does not mean that exercising is useless for weight loss. It is important for overall health, and you can shed a few kilos in the process. The problem is that it is not as effective as a solution to burn extra calories as you may be led to believe.

Not Enough Protein

If you want to shed a few kilos, you need to get enough protein into your system. In fact, protein is useful in helping you lose weight in many ways. It can suppress your appetite, make you feel full, boost your metabolic rate, decrease your calorie intake, and protect your muscle mass during weight loss.

According to a 12-day study, participants ate a diet with 30% of its calories coming from protein and they consumed on average about 575 fewer calories a day compared to a diet with 15% of its calorie coming from protein (NCBI: 23221572). Another review found that higher-protein diets that contain 0.6 to 0.8 grams of protein per pound may benefit appetite control and body composition ((NCBI: 25926512).

So, you should consider optimizing your weight loss by making sure that your diet is rich in protein.

Not Enough Fiber

A low-fiber diet tends to hamper your weight loss effort as well. Some studies suggest that viscous fiber, which is a type of soluble fiber, helps reduce your appetite by creating a gel that holds water. That way, the fiber moves slowly through your digestive tract, allowing you to feel full longer because your stomach cannot empty food as quickly.

Other research shows many other types of fiber that are beneficial for weight loss. Still, a review of many studies found that viscous fiber is the best when it comes to reducing appetite and calorie intake compared to other types of fiber (NCBI: 21676152).

When your total fiber intake is high, some of the calories in the food in mixed meals are not absorbed. According to some researchers, doubling your daily fiber intake can result in up to 130 fewer calories being absorbed into your body, meaning that you can increase the fiber content in your meal and you may absorb fewer calories although you eat the same amount of food (NCBI: 9109608).

Too Much Fat on Low-Carb Diet

Ketogenic diet and low-carb diet is not for everyone, even if they may be effective for weight loss. It all boils down to the fact that our bodies respond differently to even the same diet regimen. Studies show that those kinds of diet may reduce appetite, therefore resulting in lower calorie intake. Still, many low-carb or ketogenic diets introduce unlimited amounts of fat into the body if it means that the resulting appetite suppression can keep calories low enough for effective weight loss.

The problem here is that not many people know when to stop eating when they are on this diet because the fat is not very filling. So, the body does not receive a strong enough signal as you eat. Therefore, by the time you feel full, you may already be consuming too many calories which surpassed the calorie deficit you are trying to create.

If your food or beverage has a lot of fat and you are not losing weight, consider cutting back on the fat and see how it works.

Frequent Eating

You may be told that, in order to keep your metabolism up, you need to eat every few hours to prevent hunger. The problem here is that this leads to an excessive amount of calories being consumed and you would not feel full in the process, which paves way for overeating.

Moreover, there is another misconception floating about blood sugar level. Basically, it claims that if you do not eat, your blood sugar level will drop significantly to a dangerously low level which may result in death. Again, this is false. You do not need to look for more proof beyond survivors who managed to survive many days without eating. They survived without eating several days, you most certainly will survive 6 to 72 hours.

In a study, it is found that men who consume 3 meals within 36 hours experience a decrease in blood sugar levels and hunger while having a relatively high metabolic rate and feelings of fullness compared to men who eat 14 times over the same period of time (NCBI: 22719910).

There is also a misconception about the suggestion that you should eat breakfast every morning, regardless of appetite. According to a study, people who skip breakfast consume more calories at lunch compared to when they'd eaten breakfast. However, throughout the day, they consumed roughly 400 fewer calories (NCBI: 23672851). While it is true that your body has nothing to digest for the whole eight hours of your sleeping, that does not mean that breakfast is any more important than any other meal. You can certainly skip breakfast. There is no scientific proof that breakfast is the most important meal of the day.

You can consider trying out a different eating pattern known as intuitive eating. Here, you eat whenever your body tells you when it is hungry. Eating when and only when you are hungry seems to be the key to successful weight loss. Still, that does not mean you should allow yourself to get too hungry. It is better to have some healthy snacks than to become starving, which can result in overeating and poor food choices.

Setting Unrealistic Expectations

It is important to have clear weight loss and other health-related goals and plans to keep you motivated and track your progress. However, your goal should be realistic and attainable as well. Unrealistic expectations can work against you.

Researchers went over a huge amount of data from many weight loss center programs and they reported that overweight and obese women tend to drop out of a program after 6 to 12 months, although they expected to lose the most weight (NCBI: 16339128).

So, when you are creating your own weight loss goals, ensure that your expectations are at a more realistic and modest level. If anything, it is actually better to set a low bar first and then work your way up from there. It is more motivating for you if you see that you have achieved one goal after another, especially if you got a better result than you expected. It is better to overcome a modest hurdle and be motivated than to be discouraged by not reaching an ambitious goal. A 10% drop in weight in one year is realistic, and such a goal can prevent you from getting discouraged and improve your chances of success.

Not Tracking Your Food

Another common mistake people make is that they may be eating more calories than they think to create a calorie deficit. Eating nutritious food is a viable strategy, but this is not enough. You need to know how many calories you put into your body.

If you do not know the nutrition value of the food you eat, you may not be getting the right amount of protein, fiber, carbs, and fat to optimize your weight loss. Some studies show that tracking what you eat can give you a clearer picture of your calorie and nutrient consumption, not to mention providing accountability (NCBI: 18617080).

Moreover, many online tracking sites and mobile applications also allow you to put in your daily exercise and calculate your total calorie intake.

How to Avoid Eating Late at Night

Sometimes, you have the urge to eat late at night even though you are not really hungry. Night-time eating can cause you to eat more calories, leading to weight gain. This can be a real problem when you are at the end of your 72-hour fasting regimen. So, what can you do to avoid this?

Identify the Cause

Some people eat the largest meal in the evening or during the night. If you wish to change this habit, find out why you are doing it in the first place. In some cases, night-time eating can be the result of eating too few calories during the day, which happens to be one of the fasting mistakes we have covered in this book. This leads to ravenous hunger at night. In other cases, it can be caused by habit or boredom.

Some eating disorders may also lead to night-time eating such as binge eating disorder, and night eating syndrome. These two disorders are characterized by different eating patterns and behaviors, but they have the same negative effects on your health.

In both of them, people use food to cope with sadness, anger, or frustration, and they tend to eat even when they are not hungry. Binge eaters are also known to eat very large amounts of food in a sitting and feel powerless to stop themselves as they are eating.

Identify the Triggers

In addition to finding out the cause, you need to find which pattern of events lead you to eat at night. People turn to food for many reasons, but if you do not feel hungry and find yourself eating at night, think of the things that lead up to it. You may find a pattern, and they tend to not involve hunger. To find a pattern, you should keep a "food and mood" diary where you track what you eat and what you are feeling. You should see patterns, which helps you work on breaking any negative cycles of behavior.

Routine

If you are overeating because you do not eat enough during the day, find a routine that you can follow. Having a structure of eating and sleeping helps you spread your food intake more evenly throughout the day so you do not feel as hungry at night.

You should also get a good sleep as well because it helps maintain your food intake and weight. A lack of sleep and short sleep duration are linked to higher calorie intake and poor-quality diets. Over time, poor sleep can even increase your risk of obesity and other diseases.

So, have a set time of eating and sleeping so you can separate these two activities, especially if you tend to wake up at night to eat.

Seek Emotional Support

As we mentioned earlier, some people eat to cope with their feelings. If you think that you are having this problem, then you should seek professional help. A professional may be able to help you identify your triggers and implement a treatment plan. Most of the time, this involves cognitive behavioral therapy that has been effective in dealing with many eating disorders. In addition, you should create an emotional support network to help you manage negative emotions.

De-Stress

Anxiety and stress are two of the main reasons why people eat even though they are not hungry. In addition to seeking emotional support and professional help, there are plenty of relaxation tricks out there that you can try.

Relaxation techniques can be as simple as breathing exercises, meditation, hot baths, stretching, gentle exercises, or yoga.

Remove Junk Food

If you find that eating junk food at night is a problem, consider removing it from your house. If these things are harder to get, you are less likely to eat them. After all, who would drive to the nearest fast food chain at 2 in the morning just to grab some chicken wings?

Instead, replace the junk food with healthy snacks so even if you do eat at night, you would eat healthily. It could be fruits, berries, plain yogurt, and cottage cheese. They are very filling so you would not overeat.

Chapter 12: Conclusion

That is everything you need to know about intermittent fasting. Thank you for reading this far and we hope that this book has been educational for you.

Intermittent fasting is meant to be blended seamlessly into your daily routine so there is no need to stress too much about it. Just take your time and stick to what works best for you, and you will lose weight sustainably over time. Intermittent fasting is a very healthy way to lose weight as it is natural for our bodies.

By following the tips in this book, you should be well on your way to lose weight and become slim and healthy. We wish you good luck on your endeavor!

Lightning Source UK Ltd.
Milton Keynes UK
UKHW032335011222
413238UK00010B/89